GINKGO: THE SMART HERB

ALSO BY JONATHAN ZUESS

The Natural Prozac Program:
How to Use St. John's Wort, the Antidepressant Herb

The Wisdom of Depression:
A Guide to Understanding and
Curing Depression Using Natural Medicine

GINKGO

The Smart Herb

JONATHAN ZUESS, M.D.

THREE RIVERS PRESS

New York

Published by Three Rivers Press, a division of Crown Publishers, Inc., 201 East 50th Street, New York, New York 10022.
Member of the Crown Publishing Group.

Random House, Inc. New York, Toronto, London, Sydney, Auckland
www.randomhouse.com

THREE RIVERS PRESS and colophon are trademarks of
Crown Publishers, Inc.

Printed in the United States of America

Library of Congress Cataloging-in-Publication Data
Zuess, Jonathan.
    Ginkgo : the smart herb / Jonathan Zuess.
       p.   cm.
    Includes index.
    1. Ginkgo—Therapeutic use.   I. Title.
  RM666.G489Z84   1998
  615'.3257—dc21   98-8680
                                        CIP

ISBN 0-609-80362-X

10 9 8 7 6 5 4 3 2 1

First Edition

To Dion and Nachshon—for the future.
To R. Ayla Grafstein, Steve Klemow, and Shlomo—true friends.

CONTENTS

works • Enhancing cerebral circulation •
Protecting against stress and toxins • Boosting the
brain's smart chemicals • Beyond the brain

Appendixes

IMPORTANT NOTICE

This book is not intended for use as a substitute for consultation with a qualified medical practitioner. If you have symptoms of any of the illnesses described in this book, it is essential that you see your doctor without delay. You are unique, and your diagnosis and treatment must be individualized for you by your own doctor. This book provides exciting information about ginkgo, but no book can replace the personalized care that you need.

The author or his agents will not accept responsibility for injury, loss, or damage occasioned to any person acting or refraining to act as a result of material in this book, whether or not such injury, loss, or damage is due in any way to any negligent act or omission, breach of duty, or default on the part of the author or his agents.

For the sake of privacy, the names of the patients described in this book, and the details that might identify them, have been changed.

GINKGO: THE SMART HERB

Introduction

THE EARTH'S OWN SMART DRUG
AND ANTI-AGING REMEDY

For centuries the Taoist monks of Japan and China have revered ginkgo tea as an elixir of longevity and an aid to clearing their minds and deepening their meditations. They grew ginkgo in their monastery gardens for these purposes. Now we know there is scientific truth behind their sacred tradition.

A major study published in the *Journal of the American Medical Association* has recently proven ginkgo to be effective in relieving the symptoms of dementia, bringing this ancient medicine into prominence in the United States. Many other recent studies have shown that it works to improve mental performance in healthy people as well. It boosts memory, alertness, information processing, and reaction time. And yes, it can actually help people enter a state of heightened concentration and meditation more easily, as EEG (brain-wave) tracings demonstrate. Most remarkably, instead of stressing the brain as many stimulants do, ginkgo helps protect the brain.

Acting in several different ways at once, it shields the brain from the effects of stress, toxins, and aging.

Through ginkgo's antioxidant and gentle blood-thinning capacities, it also protects against age-related diseases throughout the body. Dozens of studies have shown that it helps prevent degenerative conditions of the heart, arteries, eyes, ears, and other organs. There is evidence that it can cure impotence and even prevent cancer. It is truly a broad-spectrum anti-aging remedy.

As large-scale studies with thousands of patients have proven, ginkgo is far safer than synthetic drugs. With all these benefits it's little wonder that ginkgo is already the number-one-selling herb in Europe and is actually one of the most-prescribed medicines of any type by European doctors. The German federal health commission lists it among the herbs deemed "safe and effective," and German and French M.D.'s have relied on it extensively for the last thirty years.

In *Ginkgo: The Smart Herb,* we'll trace the story of ginkgo from its beginnings in the traditions of prehistoric Far Eastern shamans, through to the very latest studies that have made even conventional American M.D.'s start prescribing it. You'll discover all about how to use ginkgo safely and effectively for yourself. You'll find out where to buy it and which forms are best, as well as how much to take, how often, and the results you can expect. You'll learn how you can grow and prepare it yourself. Importantly, there's also complete information on the side effects and on who should *not* use ginkgo.

Chapter 1

HOW GINKGO CAN HELP YOU

Icho, the Tree of Wisdom and Longevity

In the glow of an autumn afternoon, the venerable head monk Ikkyu Moritake pauses on the path in the monastery garden. He has come to his favorite spot, a stand of sacred icho trees on the bank of a stream. Soon they will be drawing their strength from their leaves, he muses, transmuting them to pale yellow and allowing them to fall, in preparation for the winter. But the trees themselves have hardly changed since the day he entered the monastery as an initiate some seventy years ago. The old monks in those days told him that the trees were already a thousand years old. Some said they would live forever. This is because the trees are so much in tune with the Tao, they explained, the mysterious harmony that is the source of all things.

A warm breeze from the east hushes through the stately limbs of the icho trees and stirs Ikkyu's robes. He smiles to himself as he casts his mind back through the years. He remembers his youth spent secretly questioning all the things he heard from his elders. He was skeptical of the reverence the monks and the villagers alike had for icho. He did not understand why they prized the tea they made from its leaves, telling him it was an elixir of longevity and wisdom. Now he knows well the reasons for their beliefs.

He knows that his step is lighter, his mind clearer, and his meditation deeper when he takes the tea. So for the last thirty years, he has drunk the tangy, slightly bitter green tea in the mornings and in the evenings. Yes, these trees that the monks tended so carefully really are a source of healing.

There is wisdom in the ancient ways, he knows.

Philip's Story

Philip takes the exit off I-7 and weaves through the morning traffic on Sixteenth Street. He drains his OJ and sticks the styrofoam cup back in its holder. So much for breakfast. He isn't taking any chances about being late today. He has a meeting with a potentially important new client and was up half of last night polishing the presentation. But he still feels sharp.

What a change from last year, he thinks to himself. He has lots more energy—and he is thinking more clearly. He still has a crazy lifestyle, but now he is looking after himself. Eating right—well, at least when he can; getting more exercise; and taking ginkgo. His doctor recommended it.

Philip is lucky—his doctor is progressive and keeps up

with a wide range of journals. He's read about the latest studies on the extract of Ginkgo biloba and has started to prescribe it for his patients. Philip's doctor admitted that he was surprised that the research showed it useful for so many conditions. But once he prescribed it, he said he'd seen first-hand how effective it was.

Last year, when Philip first saw his doctor, he'd been feeling really stressed out from his work. It demands constant peak mental performance, and lately he'd just been too absent-minded and tired to concentrate well. He was getting headaches nearly every day. And he was having some cramping in his legs when he walked, which was becoming a nuisance.

His doctor had said his symptoms were due partly to work stress and partly to poor blood flow. Philip had widespread vascular disease, he said, affecting not just the arteries supplying his legs but those supplying his brain and his heart muscle as well. Like many people in their fifties, Philip hadn't been looking after himself as well as he should. Without some major lifestyle changes, said the doctor, Philip would probably eventually develop a lot worse problems than just leg cramps. So along with exercise and nutritional recommendations, his doctor prescribed ginkgo extract. He said it had been proven to help with vascular disease and could also rev up brain functioning.

Philip was a skeptic about herbs. Didn't they have something to do with crystals, and fairies, and things like that? Shrugging his shoulders, though, he agreed to try the stuff.

He took one capsule twice a day—that's all there was to it.

For the first week he didn't notice much. Maybe he did feel a little more alert, and maybe concentrating was a little easier. But he certainly didn't feel any side effects, he reasoned, so he might as well keep taking it.

Then, at a board meeting during the second week, he had checked his watch and suddenly been amazed. He'd been sitting in the meeting for over two hours, yet he still felt fresh and able to pay full attention. Usually he'd be half-asleep by then, even with a couple of cups of java on board. That's when ginkgo really started to impress him.

Beginning in the third week, his walking became easier, too. He could go three or four times as far before his legs got tired. Things like his friends' phone numbers, or where he left his keys, didn't slip his mind as they used to. His headaches totally disappeared. Over the next few months, his energy level continued to increase. He felt more able to exercise, adding to his recovery.

Now, after a year on ginkgo, Philip feels like he's a year younger—or five years. Even though he's working just as many hours, it's a lot easier.

Like the millions of Europeans who take ginkgo every day, Philip has discovered for himself the healing power of this ancient herb. Now that studies have recently been published in even some of the most conservative medical journals, more and more doctors are prescribing it. It's a medication like no other—a brain enhancer and an antioxidant that can not only treat the diseases of aging but slow down the process of aging itself. As you'll discover in this book, ginkgo really is the smart herb.

Who Will Benefit from Using Ginkgo?

Ginkgo is not for the elderly alone. In studies that are as high quality as those conducted on medicines of all types, ginkgo extract has been proven to help people think smarter—regardless of whether they're young or old, sick or healthy.[1] Researchers classify it as a broad-spectrum *nootropic,* which means "mind enhancer." It improves memory, alertness, and the ability to think clearly.

Ginkgo is ideal for people under chronic stress who need to maintain peak mental performance. It boosts both memory and ability to process information, while decreasing the effects of stress on the brain. It's not a stimulant, though. Stimulants can add to the stress on the brain by forcing it to work more rapidly, and then cause fatigue and depressed mood with prolonged use. They don't improve memory, either. Ginkgo, in contrast, actually protects the brain from chemical breakdowns and damage due to stress.[2] It increases the circulation of blood to the brain, supplying it with more oxygen and nutrients and washing away metabolic wastes.[3] It reduces fatigue and has mood-elevating properties, especially with long-term use. In fact, its antistress and antidepressant effects are so strong that it can cure depressed people who are unresponsive to standard antidepressant medications.[4]

Ginkgo can also help people who need just an occasional quick memory boost, as when they're taking an exam or facing a difficult job situation. Studies of young people prove that it really works, even after a single dose.[5] Nor are these merely placebo effects. The studies were double-blind and placebo-controlled, meaning that during the tests neither the subjects nor the laboratory personnel knew whether they were using ginkgo or an inactive placebo. When the results were analyzed, the subjects taking ginkgo had consistently superior effects.

Research on brain waves (EEGs) shows that ginkgo can amplify whatever kind of waves the brain is producing.[6] That means that whatever activity you're doing, it can help you use your mind more effectively. If you're concentrating on a math problem, you'll concentrate more powerfully; if you're trying to remember something, you'll remember it more clearly; and so on. Tests also show that it increases the speed with which you process information and quickens your response time.[7]

People taking ginkgo have more beta waves in their EEGs—the kind of brain waves that occur when you're alert and thinking clearly. Ginkgo also enhances the production of alpha waves—the waves that correspond to deep, clear thought, found in people in advanced meditative states. In addition it helps reduce the number of theta waves—the kind you get when you're feeling fuzzy-headed or mentally dull.[8] All this explains why ginkgo leaf tea has traditionally been used as an aid to meditation.

But as traditional Chinese monks and herbalists know, ginkgo does more than enhance the mind. It's also a broad-spectrum anti-aging remedy. It protects against the effects of aging on the entire body. Its antioxidant effects prevent damage to our cells from toxins, radiation, pollution, inflammation, and stress—all of which have become more and more difficult to avoid in today's world. It has been proven to help prevent or treat degenerative diseases of the brain, heart, blood vessels, eyes, ears, and other organs. It can reverse impotence and even help prevent cancer.[9]

People with hardening of the arteries, or atherosclerosis, will benefit from the way ginkgo improves circulation throughout the body. Unlike other such medications, ginkgo has a preferential effect on areas that aren't receiving enough blood flow. So it effectively relieves leg cramps due to poor blood flow (also known as intermittent claudication) and angina, among other conditions. It's a gentle blood thinner, too, meaning it should reduce the risk of heart attack or stroke.[10]

Modern research has validated many of ginkgo's other traditional uses as well. For example, Chinese physicians have long treated asthma with ginkgo tea. We now know that ginkgo does indeed decrease bronchial spasm and inflammation in people with asthma, helping them breathe more easily.[11] It's also been proven to be a gentle yet powerful treatment for many other common diseases—including allergies, PMS, and diabetes.[12] It can also boost immunity and stimulate wound healing.[13]

This is impressive stuff. Ginkgo can do so many different things that it's hard to believe it's all true. After all, in Western medicine we're used to drugs that have only one specific purpose. We use an antibiotic for an infection, for instance, or an antacid to treat heartburn. When people claim something is a cure-all, we're rightly suspicious of it. So doctors from all over the world have looked at these ginkgo studies with incredulity and asked, "Are they all for real?" In several major journals they've carefully reviewed and reevaluated the studies, breaking down the data and taking a good hard look at it all again.[14] But ginkgo has come through stronger than ever.

How does it do it? Unlike synthetic drugs, ginkgo contains scores of different active ingredients.[15] For example, *ginkgolides,* a major group of chemicals in ginkgo, act to thin the blood, increase blood flow, and decrease inflammation. *Bioflavonoids,* on the other hand, are antioxidants, protecting cells from attack by toxic chemicals. Many other types of healing compounds are also found in ginkgo—some not yet fully understood.

Interestingly, when you break down ginkgo into its individual components, no single one of them seems to have the ability to do all these things. To get the best effect, you need to use the whole, unpurified extract, like the kind sold in health food stores. The drug companies, with their refined synthetic products, will never be able to come up with anything as versatile as ginkgo. Ginkgo does far more than any synthetic drug could ever do.

What You Can Expect

We now have data from studies with thousands of patients who have taken ginkgo, so we have a very clear idea of what you can expect from it. First of all, ginkgo starts working rapidly. If you take the right dose, it can boost your mental performance within an hour.[16] Interestingly, you may not even notice at first that your memory and mental sharpness have increased. In experiments, even though the tests results clearly showed that people taking ginkgo were remembering more and thinking faster, they themselves didn't feel any different.[17] Perhaps that's because our own mental performance is hard to quantify without the objective proof of lab tests.

Studies also tell us that the *full* effects of ginkgo take at least two to four weeks to come on.[18] The active ingredients need time to build up in your body, and your brain needs time to respond to them, producing the therapeutic effect. In fact, in some studies the subjects' mental functioning continued to improve for an entire year.[19] This is probably because ginkgo is capable of healing and revitalizing areas of the brain that are not working properly, because of injuries, poor blood flow, or other factors. If you keep a diary and use the simple mental exercise that I describe in chapter 8, you'll be able to objectively log your own improvement with ginkgo.

You may notice that with ginkgo you have an increased ability to keep your train of thought focused and to engage in sustained conversation about complex topics. You may feel more alert in general, too. If you're giving ginkgo to a person with dementia, expect a moderate and gradual improvement in their abilities to remember things, stay attentive, and interact socially in appropriate ways. They may well also experience some improvement in their ability to look after their own needs, like grooming themselves.

You're also likely to notice an increase in the amount of energy you feel. This may be related to ginkgo's mood-boosting effects. In many studies it had the unexpected bonus of relieving headaches, dizziness, and anxiety.[20]

Ginkgo will also improve your blood circulation. If you have chronically cold hands and feet, for instance, they will probably start to feel warmer. And if you have a disease of the cardiovascular system, like leg cramps or angina, you may also experience significant relief. (See chapter 4 for more information.)

If you have asthma, you are likely to notice fewer problems with late-night shortness of breath and coughing. Hay fever and other allergic conditions can also improve, as you'll discover in chapter 5. Sufferers of PMS will also notice less fluid retention, which can relieve many of their symptoms.

One of ginkgo's other remarkable effects is protection from the effects of radiation—including the ultraviolet radiation in sunlight.[21] You can expect to sunburn less easily and to recover quicker if you are burned. Ginkgo acts synergistically with other antioxidants, like vitamin C and E, so you'll get an increased effect from them.[22] You can even decrease your dose of other antioxidants and still get the same benefits.

As for side effects, the vast majority of people taking ginkgo have none at all. It's far safer than almost any other medication. Rarely it can cause mild stomach upset, headache, and skin rashes. To avoid these effects, you should observe a few basic precautions in taking it. For instance, people who suffer from migraines may need a lower dose. It may interact with certain medications, too. (See chapters 7 and 9 for more information.)

Ginkgo's remarkable safety and effectiveness put it in a class of its own. It seems almost tailor made to help relieve the stresses and treat the diseases of modern life. So you can expect another thing from ginkgo: it is going to absolutely rock the medical industry here in the United States. It's already done it in Europe, becoming one of the biggest-selling medications of any type.

Even though we're only now starting to discover ginkgo's effectiveness, the shamans and herbalists of Asia find nothing surprising about it. In the next chapter we'll look at how ginkgo has been a trusted part of a great healing tradition since before the beginnings of recorded history.

Chapter 2

WHAT IS GINKGO?

Not far from ground zero in Hiroshima—the epicenter of the atomic bomb detonation—there is a national park dedicated to two things. First, it is a monument to that horrific, world-changing event. But it also commemorates a quieter, yet equally awesome occurrence. A tree grows in this park—a remarkable tree. It alone, out of all the plants in the area, survived the explosion. In the spring of 1946 it actually sent out tender new shoots. The tree became a symbol of rebirth and hope to the entire Japanese nation. It's still growing there today. It's a ginkgo tree.

Ginkgo biloba has often been planted in inner-city areas around the world, since its hardiness allows it to withstand polluted air and soil that would kill other trees. It grows up to forty meters tall and has heavy, gangly-looking limbs. Its leaves are a deep green color, thick and tough-textured, and are fan-shaped, with two lobes. The species is dioecious, meaning it has separate male and female trees. The male trees produce abundant pollen, and the females produce fruits that look a lot like apricots. There's no mistaking the fruits, though—they smell like a cross between rancid butter and vomit. They can give you a rash if you handle them. Botanists have long been puzzled about why the ginkgo should produce such strange fruit.

When you learn about ginkgo, you'll be left shaking your head, too. The whole species just shouldn't exist—it's too improbable. But sometimes truth really is stranger than fiction. Let me take you on a journey now, back 200 million years, to where the story of ginkgo begins—deep in the early Jurassic period.

The Real Jurassic Park *Story*

Once there were some trees that decided they needed animals. Mammals—those awkward, rodentlike creatures who incubate their young within their own bodies instead of laying eggs like any decent reptile—had just appeared on the scene. These odd little mammals were hungry, too. They gobbled up all the seeds, fruits, and nuts that the trees could produce. It was crisis time for the trees. If none of their seeds survived, no more young trees would grow. The trees rallied and tried to defend themselves. They produced thicker and harder coats around their seeds, hoping to discourage the mammals. But the animals had strong teeth to crack the coats. Nothing worked.

One tree, though, was especially wise. Instead of resisting

the little mammals, it decided to cooperate with them. Why not let the animals take home its seeds and store them in their burrows underground? Wouldn't that be a good way to have its seeds dispersed and planted? All the tree needed to do was to work out a way to discourage the animals from eating its seeds too quickly, ensuring that they would take the seeds home and plant them.

Then it worked out the solution. It would produce a nasty-tasting, toxic coat around the seeds. The coat would decay and dissolve over a period of weeks, but the seeds themselves would be big, tasty, and nutritious. (In other words, the seeds would be nuts.) The animals would love to munch on the seeds, but they wouldn't be able to eat them right away. Instead, they would have to take them home, store them underground for safekeeping, and let the coats dissolve. Then they could eat them. And since they would have to leave the buried seeds alone for such a long time, the animals would inevitably forget about some of them. Some of the seeds would be bound to survive and sprout into saplings.

In this way the tree would go into partnership with the mammals—using them to help spread its seeds far and wide.[1] The mammals would look after the needs of the tree, and the tree, in turn, would allow the mammals to eat many of its seeds.

This tree was the ancestor of the ginkgo. The solution worked well, and so the ginkgo flourished. It spread throughout the cool northern forests of the Jurassic period, developing into fifty different species. Whole forests of ginkgo appeared. With its special relationship with mammals, it hardly noticed the disappearance of the dinosaurs. While other tree species came and went, ginkgos were so successful that they survived unchanged for literally millions of years— far longer than any other tree. Individual ginkgo trees themselves were incredibly long-lived, up to two thousand years or more. Their leaves, branches, and roots were loaded with powerful antioxidant and healing chemicals that helped the trees defy the aging process.

But then a new threat appeared on the earth, far more dangerous than mammals, dinosaurs, or old age: ice.

The Sacred Survivor

The ice ages transformed the northern forests into glacial wastelands. Animals and plants alike retreated south if they could, but many were unable to make the transition and froze in the cold, becoming extinct. Unfortunately ginkgo had one weakness: it was slow-growing. The young ginkgo trees at the southern edge of the advancing ice front were unable to mature fast enough to produce seeds before the cold caught up to them and killed them. They were unable to spread their seeds south like the other, faster-growing tree species. Forty-nine of the ginkgo species were wiped out. Only one remained, and it was in grave danger.

Long ago, though, ginkgo had made that wise decision to become partners with the mammals. Once more the decision paid off. Because now there was one very special kind of mammal on the scene—a species that could save ginkgo. This species, like the awkward rodents of the distant past, loved to eat ginkgo's nutritious seeds. It also ate the leaves in small quantities. It had discovered that the ginkgo's healing chemicals, which help the trees live so long, could also help heal its own diseases. This species had made the step from simply storing the seeds underground to intentionally planting them and cultivating ginkgo. This species was the human.

It is thought that the shamans of ancient China, long before the advent of Buddhism, were probably responsible for saving ginkgo from extinction during the ice ages. The shamans cultivated it, and later, monks gave it refuge in their monastery gardens and took it with them when they established new monasteries. The tree was sacred to them as a source of both food and medicine. They planted it also as a symbol of wisdom and centeredness. Buddhists called the tree "Buddha's fingernails" because of the shape of the leaves. The Taoists saw the yin and yang symbol in the leaves' two lobes.

A few stands of wild ginkgo have recently been discovered in remote forests in eastern China, in the provinces of Anhui, Zhejiang, and Guizhou.[2] Some scientists say these stands are escapees from monasteries. It's possible, though, that they are remnants of the ginkgos that survived the ice age outside the monasteries. Still, there is no question that Asian shamans and monks have cultivated ginkgo since prehistoric times. As we'll see, the very earliest records of Chinese medicine attest to this.

The Elixir of Emperors

Shining through a Chinese text written thousands of years ago comes wisdom from a still earlier time—from before writing even existed. The *Shennong Bencaojing (Pharmaceutical Classic of the Master of Husbandry)* may have been the first book on herbalism ever written. It is credited to the legendary Emperor Shen Nong (3494 B.C.E.) and contains a collection of healing secrets that were undoubtedly passed down from prehistoric shamans. In this earliest record of Chinese medicine, we find a discussion of the use of ginkgo leaves for boosting memory and treating breathing problems like asthma and bronchitis. They used the leaves to make tea or soaked them in rice wine to make an alcohol-based extract.

Throughout history Chinese medical texts added to the list of uses for ginkgo. The leaves were used externally, as a poultice to help heal wounds and to treat sun damage (freckles), and internally, to improve circulation to the limbs in cases of frostbite. The fruit pulp was used as a treatment for infections and intestinal parasites. All of these uses now have scientific data that prove that they really work.

Chinese physicians, who preferred dietary treatments to medicines, also started to prescribe ginkgo seeds. Modern analysis has found that the seeds do indeed contain low concentrations of many of the same active ingredients as the leaves. They also contain lots of nutritious complex carbohydrates and monounsaturated fatty acids, making them a cross between a food and a medicine.

In traditional Chinese medicine ginkgo seeds are classified as a "kidney yang tonic," meaning they can increase energy in the urinary and sexual organs. They're used to treat impotence, bed-wetting, and bladder problems. They're also good for treating disorders of the ear, like deafness. As you'll discover in this book, modern medicine is just now beginning to discover for itself the power of ginkgo to treat things like impotence and ear disorders.

You can find ginkgo nuts for sale in Chinese grocery stores today, in cans labeled "white nut." You can also collect the nuts that fall from trees in public parks, as some Chinese people do here in the United States. The nuts have to be cooked before you can eat them—they're toxic if eaten raw. Don't eat the fruits, either; they'll irritate your stomach and intestines. The ginkgo tree intended them to do this when it developed them millions of years ago, so that mammals would have to wait for the fruits to decompose before they could eat the nuts.

Before you cook the nuts, the fruits have to be removed. Soak them in a bucket of water for a couple of weeks, allowing them to ferment and slough off. Be careful to handle the fruits only with gloves, or you may get a rash. About 30 percent of people are allergic to them.

Ginkgo Goes West

In the early eighteenth century, a German surgeon, botanist, and adventurer by the name of Engelbert Kaempfer traveled to the Orient. He was captivated by the ginkgo trees he found there and brought seeds with him back to Europe. He mistakenly called the tree ginkyo, after the Japanese name for the fruits. Actually the Japanese term *ginkyo* came originally from the Chinese *yin guo,* which means "silver fruit" or "hill apricot." The tree itself is really called *icho,* as we now know.

Kaempfer planted the first European ginkgo in the Utrecht Botanical Garden, in what is now the Netherlands, around 1730. Europeans were fascinated with all things Oriental, and ginkgo became more and more popular. The first ginkgo tree was planted in England in 1762 and in the United States in 1784. With its hardiness against pollution and pests, ginkgo was soon recognized as an ideal ornamental tree for the streets of dirty post-Industrial Revolution cities. You can still find them today downtown in many European and American cities.

A few Westerners were aware of ginkgo's role in traditional Chinese medicine, but it was not until the 1960s that ginkgo began to be investigated and gain some acceptance among Western physicians. The initial interest came mainly from Germany and France. In these countries herbal medicine had always been considered part of mainstream medical culture, in contrast to the situation in the United States and Great Britain. In Europe conventional doctors incorporated the use of herbs into their work. For example, in German medical schools today, courses on herbal medicine are part of the normal curriculum. Eighty percent of German doctors prescribe herbs. It is thanks to the enlightened, nonpolitical attitudes of European doctors that we have scientific studies on ginkgo today. In the American system, under the political and financial stranglehold of conventional medicine, these studies would probably never have been done. Only recently, because of the huge tide of scientific evidence from Europe, have American doctors started to investigate herbal medications.

Once a standardized, concentrated extract of ginkgo became available in the 1960s, formal studies of its uses began in earnest. As the research has accumulated, the use of the extract has increased dramatically. Ginkgo is now the most frequently prescribed herb in Europe. Two thousand tons of it are sold each year, representing well over five million prescriptions. The demand for it is also increasing by 26 percent per year.[3] Here in the United States ginkgo is less well known and ranks fifth among herb sales.[4] To keep up with the growing demand, herbal companies have established large plantations of ginkgo trees on the Atlantic coast of France, in South Carolina, and in China.[5] Ginkgo is also grown commercially in Japan and South Korea. Ginkgo's ancient partnership with mammals is still paying off for it.

How Is It Prepared?

All the various ginkgo preparations used in Western medicine are prepared from the leaves. The leaves are harvested in the fall, just before they start to turn color, when their concentration of active ingredients is highest.

The leaves go through several steps before they end up in

standardized ginkgo capsules on a shelf in your health food store. First they're finely ground and left to soak in a solution of acetone and water. The active ingredients dissolve out into the liquid. This is then strained, to remove the cellulose and other solid residues. Further purification techniques are used to adjust the concentrations of the major active ingredients. The extracting liquid is then mostly removed, so that what is left is more or less a gooey green-brown syrup of active ingredients. Finally ginkgo leaf powder is added as a binder, and it's packaged in capsules or gel tabs. Most of the scientific research on ginkgo has been done using standardized extracts like these.

Ginkgo is also available in nonstandardized preparations, which are less processed. For example, the leaves may simply be freeze-dried, ground up, and packaged into capsules. Or the ground leaves may be soaked in alcohol or glycerine and strained, and the unrefined liquid extract packaged for sale in small brown glass bottles. Simpler still, fresh or dried ginkgo leaves can be used to make tea. Some herbalists prefer to use these more traditional forms, despite the fact that no research has been conducted using them. In chapter 8 I discuss the pros and cons of all these various ways of using ginkgo.

Can I Harvest and Prepare It Myself?

You might have access to ginkgo trees in a public place in your own city. Finding them in an unpolluted place, however, might be more of a challenge. On the one hand, harvesting a few leaves to make tea is the simplest, most natural way to use ginkgo. On the other hand, as I'll discuss in chapter 8, it is less effective than using standardized extracts. But if you decide it's for you, you certainly can harvest and prepare it yourself. For the full details see chapter 9, on how to use ginkgo, and chapter 11, on harvesting and making your own ginkgo extract.

Chapter 3

GINKGO—THE BRAIN BOOSTER

The Truth Behind the Traditions

The wisdom of evolution, the deeply held traditions—what do these things mean to the scientist?

Not much. They're only a starting point, a hypothesis posed in the vague languages of time and legend. Instead of just accepting propositions, the scientists' task is to believe as little as possible. They have to see something for themselves before they'll accept it as true.

So when scientists came to focus their gaze on ginkgo, they were equally as willing to debunk it as they were to prove it. In study after study, they asked the same questions: Does it work? Does it work better than placebos? And if it does, how does it work?

The answers surprised them. Yes, ginkgo worked. It worked better than placebos. In fact, it worked in ways no other known medicine worked, and it helped heal conditions that no other drug helped heal. To top it all off, it did all this with virtually no side effects.

The ancient shamans of Asia and the countless other herbalists down through the millennia of Chinese history were all validated. The healing tradition had donned the white coat of science—and had received new life.

Boosting Memory

No matter how good your memory is, ginkgo can make it better. Study after study has shown it to boost memory in anyone—young or old, sick or healthy. Even though it's best known in this country for its effects on Alzheimer's disease, that's only a small part of what this nootropic can do.

In one French study, for example, ginkgo was tested on healthy young volunteers.[1] The subjects were randomly selected to be given either a single dose of ginkgo extract or a placebo pill that looked and tasted just like it. Neither the subjects nor the testing personnel knew which capsules were which—they were all marked with a secret code. In other words, it was a placebo-controlled, double-blind study—the most scientifically rigorous kind. One hour after taking the capsules, the subjects were administered a battery of tests. Then the code was broken, and the results analyzed. As expected, the results showed that the placebo had done nothing. But remarkably, after taking ginkgo, the subjects had experienced a very significant boost in their short-term memory.

The test was designed to weed out any memory-boosting that was due to a simple stimulant effect. But it showed that ginkgo is not a stimulant; instead, it produces effects quite specifically on the process of memory.

Remember, the full effect of ginkgo is believed to be produced only after a person takes it regularly for at least two weeks. So if it worked in a single dose, that would suggest ginkgo was even more effective than had been previously thought. Ever skeptical, the investigating scientists were puzzled. Could the results have just been a fluke?

So they repeated the study, using the same conditions and the same dose. The results came out the same.[2] Ginkgo wowed 'em.

Okay, we now know ginkgo works for young people. It may be useful for them when they're in a situation where every bit of short-term memory counts, like an exam. But otherwise young people's memories are usually pretty sharp. They may not need ginkgo much. Where ginkgo would clearly be more useful, you'd think, is for older people.

As we get to middle age and beyond, most of us experience a minor decrease in short-term memory. This phenomenon is considered to be a normal accompaniment of aging and is called age-associated memory impairment, or AAMI. If ginkgo could work to counteract AAMI, scientists reasoned, it would really be helping where help is needed.

The researchers set to work, and we now have several high-quality placebo-controlled, double-blind studies in this area.[3] The results are unanimous—ginkgo improves memory in AAMI. Not only that, but it can, in effect, tune up your brain—increasing the speed with which you process information.

In 1991, for instance, a group of doctors in London published the results from a study of 31 people with mild to moderate AAMI, aged fifty years and up.[4] They treated them with either ginkgo or placebo for six months. A series of tests of mental functioning showed that the patients taking ginkgo had consistent improvements both in their memory and their response time.

In 1995 psychiatrists at the University of Vienna took a closer look at how ginkgo speeds up the brain's response time.[5] In their study, 48 people with AAMI were treated with ginkgo or placebo for two months. They were then presented with visual and auditory information to which they had to respond as quickly as possible. Using highly sophisticated brain-wave and eye-movement tracking devices, the researchers measured the speed with which the subjects processed the information. Once again the subjects taking ginkgo had consistently shorter response times. They were clearly able to evaluate the information more quickly.

How do you know if you have AAMI? It's essentially just a mildly increased amount of forgetfulness. You may not even notice you have it. In fact, as scientists have discovered, a lot of older people are totally unaware they have any problems with their memory or thinking. If you perform EEGs on apparently healthy older people, for example, some of them will show abnormal brain-wave patterns. This means that they have an early stage of mental impairment totally unknown to them. A study reported in the major British journal the *Lancet* described how when ginkgo was given to people like these, their brain-wave patterns normalized. In other words, ginkgo can improve mental functioning even in people who haven't noticed that anything is wrong with them.[6]

If you do have AAMI, you can be reassured—it isn't the forerunner of dementia. As I mentioned, it's believed to be due to "normal aging." Some scientists, however, disagree, saying that AAMI is due to the cumulative effects of stress on the brain. High stress levels, they maintain, cause an increase in oxidative metabolism in the brain, as well as abnormally high levels of hormones like cortisol, both of which are known to cause damage to brain cells.

If those scientists are correct, ginkgo may be able not only to treat AAMI—but to prevent it from ever occurring. It decreases oxidation in the brain and may be able to bring into balance abnormal levels of hormones.[7]

As a result, ginkgo is appropriate for people concerned about achieving and maintaining maximum brain power for their whole lives. It's especially good for those who are just beginning to experience deterioration in their mental performance.[8] It can slow the process down, stop it, and probably even reverse it.

We've seen how ginkgo can boost the brain power of healthy people. Now let's take a look at how it does against the ultimate challenge for any nootropic: dementia.

Dementia: The Ultimate Challenge

"You can't treat dementia." That's what I was taught in medical school. Or, at least, the professors said, you can't make demented people remember things or think clearly again; all you can do is try to help them cope with the inexorable loss of their higher intellectual powers. After all, brain cells don't grow back, and that's that.

But the professors were wrong. We know now that you can treat dementia. You can improve demented people's memory, alertness, and ability to think clearly. You can even slow the course of the illness and possibly prevent it in the first place. The last fifteen years or so have seen a major change in our understanding of dementia, and we've begun to discover effective ways to treat it. Some of the medications we're discovering to be helpful are ones with which conventional doctors have long been familiar—like estrogen and non-steroidal anti-inflammatory drugs (NSAIDs). Others are newer synthetic drugs, like tacrine and donazepril. But still others have previously been found only in the pharmacopaeia of natural healers—like vitamin E and, now, ginkgo.

Ginkgo is a broad-spectrum antidementia medicine. It works in many different ways simultaneously. It doesn't treat only the commonest type of dementia, Alzheimer's disease. It treats the next most common type, too, called vascular dementia (often referred to as multi-infarct dementia). These two types of dementia account for the vast majority of all cases.

In a study published in the *Journal of the American Medical Association* in 1997, doctors in New York, Boston, and Los Angeles compared ginkgo with a placebo in 309 patients with either Alzheimer's disease or vascular dementia.[9] They were randomly divided into two groups—one group to receive standardized ginkgo extract daily (40 mg three times a day) and the other to receive the placebo. The pills all looked and tasted the same, and no one was told which pills they were receiving. After fifty-two weeks of treatment, the results were analyzed. As expected, the group receiving the placebo had not done very well, and tests showed considerable deterioration in their mental functioning. The group receiving ginkgo, on the other hand, had had no deterioration at all—in fact, they had actually had an *improvement* in their mental functioning. Put simply, ginkgo had halted or even reversed the progression of their illness. The extract worked for both Alzheimer's disease and vascular dementia.

These kinds of results are not at all unusual for ginkgo. The American doctors in that study were really only confirming the results of previous European studies. For instance, in 1996, German psychiatrists had treated 216 patients with Alzheimer's or vascular dementia for twenty-four weeks with either ginkgo or a placebo.[10] Again, the results had been very significantly in favor of ginkgo.

Ginkgo not only improves attention and memory in people with dementia, it also helps relieve their psychological symptoms, such as depressed mood, and it enhances their ability to perform household chores and self-care.[11] Their EEGs also show fewer slower and more fast waves, reflecting the improvement in their brain functioning.[12]

As I mentioned, a few synthetic drugs have now been developed to treat dementia, too. Unfortunately, they have around ten times the incidence of side effects as ginkgo.[13] Some of their side effects are very serious, including liver and bone marrow damage. Ginkgo should definitely be the first-line treatment, with these drugs used as backups.

How Ginkgo Works

Ginkgo is the most broad-spectrum medicine for the brain that we know of. As I mentioned before, it works in many different ways at once. It can do so because it contains so many different active ingredients. No single one of them accounts for all of the extract's healing powers. Instead, they act together synergistically—creating an overall effect that is greater than the sum of the parts.

Enhancing Cerebral Circulation

One way ginkgo works is through its extraordinary ability to increase the blood flow to the brain. It makes the blood more fluid, enabling it to move through arteries, veins, and capillaries more easily.[14] It relaxes the walls of contracted blood vessels, opening them up to provide better flow.[15] These actions bring in a rich supply of oxygen and nutrients and wash away metabolic wastes. Ginkgo also improves the ability of brain cells to work in conditions of low oxygen.[16]

By enhancing cerebral circulation, ginkgo can improve many symptoms other than poor memory or concentration. Studies show it relieves headaches, dizziness, depressed mood, and anxiety and increases energy levels.[17]

Protecting Against Stress and Toxins

Ginkgo is also a potent *neuroprotective* agent; that is, it shields the brain from the ravages of stress, toxins, and aging. The bioflavonoids in ginkgo, for instance, are powerful antioxidants. Antioxidants protect cells by quenching a type of chemical reaction called free radical oxidation. Free radical oxidation causes a breakdown of cell membranes, proteins, and DNA, and interferes with cellular repair mechanisms. It plays a major role in many diseases, including Alzheimer's. It is also thought to be a major cause, if not the only cause, of aging. Since ginkgo is one of the most potent antioxidants known, it's like a natural shield against these problems.[18]

The ginkgolides add to the neuroprotective power of ginkgo.[19] They inhibit the low-grade inflammation that is part of diseases like Alzheimer's. Additionally, ginkgo strengthens the brain's blood vessels, preventing abnormal leakiness caused by toxins or diseases.[20]

Boosting the Brain's Smart Chemicals

Ginkgo may also work by altering the chemistry of the brain itself. Studies in animals suggest that it may change the brain's levels of serotonin, acetylcholine, and other "smart" chemicals, which may explain why ginkgo has such a strong antidepressant effect, too.[21] No biochemical studies have been done on humans yet, so we don't know if the animal tests are really valid. Since animals' brains are so different from humans', ginkgo probably works quite differently for them.

In addition to experiments on animals, researchers now have available many different noninjurious techniques that can be used on humans. We need to wait for them to be used before we can really be certain that ginkgo changes the chemistry of the human brain.

The issue of whether animal tests should be done at all with ginkgo is an important one. When I was researching this book, I came across a number of experiments that had been performed on animals. I considered the issue carefully for some time and finally decided not to cite their results. The main reason was that most of these studies contributed nothing significant to our understanding of ginkgo. The few that did provide useful information, like the ones I alluded to above, could have been replaced by painless studies of humans. And some of the animal studies were very cruel indeed. I am one of a growing number of physicians who believe that most animal experiments are unjustified and unethical. In appendix 1 I discuss further my rationale for not citing them.

Beyond the Brain

Even if we don't have the final answer on all the ways that ginkgo works on the brain, we do know one thing for certain: it really works. The fact is, even a lot of the synthetic medications that conventional doctors use today have less good evidence to back them up.

Ginkgo does a lot more than protect and heal the brain, though. As we'll see in the next chapter, what sets it unmistakably apart from synthetic medications is its remarkable versatility. Quite simply, no other nootropic—and no other medication of any type—can equal it.

Chapter 4

GINKGO—THE LONGEVITY TONIC

The Elixir of Youth

The ancient Chinese emperors were obsessed with it. They employed alchemists full time who worked away day and night at their furnaces, heating egg-shaped concoctions of mercury and lead that they believed would be transformed into the elixir of youth. To them, the transmutation of base metals, the perfection of the soul, and the immortality of the body were all bound up in the same vortex of cosmic forces.

In a different way contemporary Westerners are obsessed with the elixir of youth, too. But now our alchemists wear white coats. Using the instruments of science, we've dissected the problem of aging, looking ever deeper into our cells and into what makes us work. We've discovered how our biological building blocks—our genes and our chemistry—are themselves stamped with the imprint of our mortality.

The first major theory of aging says that the whole process

is built into our genes. Even if we remained a hundred percent healthy throughout our lives, this theory says, we could live only a certain number of years before our programmed allotment was used up. No one is certain exactly how many years are inscribed into our genes, but many scientists believe it may be 120 or more. It's only the diseases we develop from poor lifestyle or other factors, they say, that stop us from reaching our potential life span.

The second major theory of aging says that aging isn't programmed into us at all and that it's not inevitable. Instead, this theory says, aging is due to the accumulation of rancid fats throughout the body. These fats, called peroxidized lipids, cause cells to break down and die. They're formed through free radical oxidation, a chemical reaction mentioned in the previous chapter. This reaction occurs in any situation where you're exposed to oxidative stress, such as in many chronic illnesses, exposure to toxic chemicals, or even under severe emotional stress. A diet high in damaged fats, such as those produced by frying or broiling meat, or any fats that have been altered, like those found in margarine and shortening, also greatly increases free radical oxidation in the body. Antioxidants, on the other hand, decrease it.

This is where ginkgo comes in. It's one of the most powerful antioxidants known, stopping lipid peroxidation and putting the brakes on aging. So if you believe in the second theory of aging, ginkgo is the medicine for you. But even if the first theory is the right one and aging is preprogrammed into our genes and inevitable, ginkgo can still help. It prevents, treats, and can even reverse many of the diseases that occur as we get older. It can turn around arterial and heart disease, age-related blindness, ringing in the ears, impotence, and aging of the skin, and it may even prevent cancer. If those diseases are healed, there's no reason why we wouldn't reach our maximum potential life span—maybe 120 years or more.

Let's take a closer look now at exactly how ginkgo can do all these things.

An Unclogger of Arteries

It's public enemy number one. Atherosclerosis, or hardening of the arteries, is the hit man behind about half of all deaths in Western countries. It used to affect older people only. But these days doctors hardly bat an eye when a person in their forties or even their thirties is brought into the ER with the tragic results of atherosclerosis: a heart attack or a stroke.

We all know the causes. Smoking, diets high in fat and cholesterol, and lack of regular exercise and relaxation are some of the biggies. According to some experts like Dr. Dean Ornish, lack of intimacy with others is another major factor.[1] Recently conventional doctors have come to accept what naturopaths have been saying for decades—that vitamin deficiencies (like folate and B6 deficiencies, which cause increased serum homocysteine, a promoter of atherosclerosis, and vitamin C and E deficiencies), and the use of synthetic fats like margarine, are also behind our current epidemic.

Obviously, then, you can do a lot to prevent atherosclerosis. If you have it, you have many effective options for treating it, and even reversing it, apart from the drugs and the bypass your cardiologist might recommend. One of the great things about natural methods of healing is that not only do they offer help in curing disease, but unlike the methods of conventional medicine, the very same alternative methods can prevent disease, too. A healthy diet and lifestyle, for instance, can both cure and prevent diseases of the heart and arteries. Ginkgo extract is another good example—it's both preventive and curative.

By acting on the cardiovascular system in several different ways at once, ginkgo can not only prevent disease but, if you already have it, can help improve blood flow and decrease symptoms. Through its antioxidant effects, it can protect blood vessels from the effects of a toxic diet, stress, and aging.[2] It increases the ability of cells in the walls of blood vessels to take up nutrients, helping them fight damage due to atherosclerosis.[3] It can help lower cholesterol and fat levels in the blood, too.[4]

One of the most remarkable qualities of ginkgo is its preferential effect on areas of the body that are not getting enough blood flow.[5] It relaxes the walls of small arteries, allowing a healthy supply of blood to previously blocked-off tissues and clearing out toxins.[6] Few other medications can do this.

Many people who have heart disease, high blood pressure, cholesterol problems, or diabetes also have abnormally sticky or viscous blood, putting them at risk for artery blockages. They have too much of the clotting protein *fibrinogen,* and their platelets, the tiny cell fragments in the blood that are in charge of blood clotting, are abnormally sticky. Ginkgo can reverse these problems, improving the fluidity of the blood, and decreasing the risk of abnormal clotting.[7] It does this by reducing the effects of platelet activating factor (PAF), a chemical in the body responsible for causing blood clots. This in turn can help prevent heart attack and stroke.

Coronary heart disease is one of the end results of a long-term buildup of atherosclerotic plaque. It causes a decreased flow of blood to the heart muscle, usually experienced as chest pain on exertion (angina). In a 1996 study ginkgo extract was shown to effectively relieve angina and improve abnormal electrocardiograms (EKGs) in these patients.[8]

Atherosclerosis can also decrease the blood flow to the legs. When it does, people have a symptom called *intermittent claudication*—cramping pain in the legs when walking. Like heart disease, this problem is very common among older people. The first line of treatment is simple: stop smoking, and start walking regularly. But for many people that's not enough. In these cases conventional American doctors sometimes prescribe a drug called Trental (pentoxifylline). It's only modestly effective, however, and the current opinion is that its cost and inconvenience rarely make it worthwhile.[9] But for decades European doctors have had a better solution for intermittent claudication: ginkgo. A large amount of research proves that ginkgo provides effective relief for this disorder.[10]

In a very high-quality study in 1996, for example, 60 patients with intermittent claudication were randomly assigned to receive either ginkgo extract or placebo.[11] They were placed on a steep treadmill, and the distance they could walk before the cramping in their legs started was measured. After two months of treatment, the patients receiving ginkgo were able to walk three times farther than those receiving the placebo. After six months, they could walk five times farther.

In severe cases of claudication, the pain occurs even at rest. When it gets this bad, there is often no option left other than surgery—a graft to the arteries in the leg, or amputation. But ginkgo can help even in these cases. In a study from France, treatment with ginkgo gave significant relief to patients with pain at rest.[12]

In all, sixteen controlled trials have been done on the use of ginkgo for intermittent claudication. All except one have shown that ginkgo is highly effective, with few or no side effects.[13]

We've seen how cardiovascular disease is the number-one disease of aging, and how ginkgo is an ideal treatment for it. Now let's look at how it stacks up against number two: cancer.

Cancer Prevention

It's more feared than any other kind of illness. Most people don't realize, though, that the majority of cancers are preventable—the National Cancer Institute estimates the figure at 80 percent.[14] Like atherosclerosis, cancer is mainly a lifestyle disease, related to preventable modern hazards like poor diet, lack of activity, chronic stress, smoking, pollutants, and radiation. The evidence is mounting that antioxidants can prevent cancer. Ginkgo probably can, too.

In the department of genetics at the University of Paris, a team of researchers have been investigating the use of ginkgo in preventing cancer.[15] They've been studying one of the highest-risk populations of all time: workers who cleaned up after the Chernobyl nuclear reactor accident. In the workers' blood they've discovered cancer-causing particles called *clastogenic factors,* similar to those discovered in the blood of A-bomb survivors. *Clastogenic* means "causing breaks in chromosomes"—the first step in the creation of a cancer.

Disturbingly, the researchers have also discovered that you don't need to have been exposed to massive amounts of radiation to have these cancer-causing factors in your blood. They can be produced by the same conditions that cause free radical oxidation—illness, toxins, stress, and eating damaged or synthetic fats. Everybody probably has some clastogenic factors in their blood.

How do you get rid of these things? You need antioxidants—and powerful ones. Ginkgo fits the bill. The University of Paris researchers therefore tested ginkgo on human blood samples that had been irradiated.[16] It cleared up the clastogenic factors nicely. Encouraged, the researchers then treated the Chernobyl workers with ginkgo extract, giving them 40 mg three times a day for two months.[17] Ginkgo reduced the clastogenic factors in their blood way down to the level of people who had never been exposed to radiation. The effect lasted for seven months after the ginkgo was stopped.

Granted, this result doesn't *prove* that ginkgo can prevent cancer, since the study wasn't long-term enough. It does strongly suggest, however, that it can.

Perhaps even more fascinating, ginkgo looks as if it may not only prevent cancer but treat it as well. Chemical analysis has shown that ginkgo contains at least nineteen types of chemicals that have anticancer effects.[18] Japanese researchers, for instance, have reported that a group of compounds from ginkgo leaves, the *long-chain phenols,* have "strong antitumor activity" against leukemia and other cancers.[19] The bio-flavonoids quercetin and kaempferol, which make up about a quarter of the weight of the standardized extracts you can purchase, are also known to have anticancer effects.[20] Ginkgolide B, too, through its immunity-boosting effects, increases the production of *tumor necrosis factor,* one of the body's own defenses against cancer.[21]

Preventing Skin Aging

Through its anticlastogenic effects, ginkgo can protect you from all sorts of radiation—including solar radiation. In a remarkable study from Germany published in 1992, ginkgo was shown to protect sunbathers from damage due to ultraviolet light rays—the kind that cause sunburn, aging of the skin, and skin cancer.[22] Other antioxidants were tested, too. Ginkgo proved itself superior to vitamin E and beta-carotene. Only selenium was better than ginkgo.

A second study looked at the details of how ginkgo protects

against skin damage due to sunlight.[23] It seems that when radiation hits the skin, free radicals are formed. These free radicals then react with fatty acids inside cells, causing them to become peroxidized. As I explained above, peroxidized lipids are believed to be a cause of the aging process. Free radicals are also clastogenic and can cause cancer. Ginkgo mops up the free radicals before they have a chance to do any damage and so prevents skin aging and cancer.

If ginkgo can protect you from ultraviolet radiation, it should also work for other kinds of radiation, like X-rays. One expert has recommended recently that anyone who is about to have X-rays taken, or who knows they will be exposed to any kind of radiation, should take a dose of ginkgo beforehand to protect themselves.[24] He also notes that ginkgo may shorten the recovery time from sunburn and reduce its pain.

Ginkgo is not a replacement for protecting your skin from the sun with long sleeves, a hat, and sunscreen, but it adds another level of protection.

Preserving Vision

It's the number-one cause of legal blindness in people over 65: macular degeneration. And it's treatable. How? Ginkgo.

Sensing light involves a complex and intense metabolic process. The cells of the macula use up more energy than any other cells in the body. The macula is a round spot right in the middle of the retina—the thin layer of cells in the back of the eyeball that senses light. The macula is at the center of our visual field, the part that sees fine detail best. Because of its high metabolic rate, the macula needs a lot of oxygen. But whenever cells use a lot of oxygen, they risk being damaged by it—oxidation. So the macula is one of the tissues most susceptible to oxidative damage in the body. When this damage goes on for a long period of time, it produces a condition called macular degeneration. People with this condition lose the ability to see things at the center of their visual field and to see details like fine print. They can't drive, either.

Until recently, there was no known treatment for the majority of people with macular degeneration. In rare cases laser surgery was effective, but most people were sent home from their ophthalmologist with advice on "low-vision aids"—a euphemism for magnifying glasses and other such things. Now we know ginkgo can help.

In a small placebo-controlled, double-blind study, patients with macular degeneration were treated with 80 mg a day of ginkgo extract.[25] After six months of treatment, they were found to have a significant improvement in their vision.

Ginkgo's antioxidant effects are probably the main reason it works for this condition. It's now been well established that antioxidants like vitamin A, E, and C can prevent macular degeneration from occurring in the first place. They also help prevent cataracts. Therefore it's likely that ginkgo can prevent these problems as well.

Ginkgo also improves blood flow in the eyes of elderly people. Studies show it can improve the vision of people with poor circulation in the eye caused by atherosclerosis or diabetes.[26] It improves both the sensitivity of the retina to light and the ability to distinguish colors.

Why is ginkgo so effective for visual problems? The eye and the brain have a very special connection. In the embryo the eyes develop as little buds growing out from the front of the brain, and they continue to share certain biochemical characteristics with the brain as they mature. That helps explain why ginkgo has an affinity for both these tissues.

Relief from Ringing in the Ears

Have you ever been to a concert or a club and noticed afterward that your ears were ringing? You've experienced briefly a disorder that many people deal with every day of their lives. Ear, nose, and throat (ENT) specialists will tell you that one of the most difficult to treat of all the maladies they encounter is tinnitus, or ringing in the ears. It can be caused by many different things, but it's usually due to long-term exposure to loud noise. Such noise damages the delicate hair cells in the organ of Corti, the structure located in the inner ear that is responsible for hearing.

Rock musicians inevitably suffer from tinnitus, and so does much of their audience. Earphones are another major source of high-intensity noise, and so is traffic noise and loud tools. The first few times the ear is exposed to loud noise, the tinnitus goes away as the ear adapts. But soon the ears aren't able to adapt any longer, and the tinnitus or hearing loss becomes permanent. Among baby boomers it has become a serious problem. It's starting to show up among Generation Xers, too, as the toll on their ears adds up.

American medical textbooks will tell you that no medication is effective in treating noise-induced tinnitus. In desperation ENT specialists here will sometimes prescribe a sedative or antidepressant for it. But in Europe ENT doctors use ginkgo—and they have good studies to back up their choice.

In one such study ENT specialists from several different clinics in France treated a total of 103 tinnitus patients with ginkgo.[27] In this placebo-controlled, double-blind study lasting thirteen months, they discovered that ginkgo improved the condition of all the patients—irrespective of how long their tinnitus had been going on, and irrespective even of its cause. Another study, this one with 259 patients, confirmed these findings.[28] Tinnitus is now one of the conditions for which the German government has approved ginkgo.

A recent small study from Sweden, however, reported no improvement with ginkgo.[29] This may have been because it only included 20 patients, and because these patients were selected because they had the most severe and longstanding cases of tinnitus that the doctors could find. Naturally they were more difficult to treat.

Ginkgo also improves other disorders of the inner ear. Vertigo, or dizziness, is one such disorder. In two separate studies, ginkgo was shown to work significantly better than placebo for it.[30] Acute deafness due to inner-ear damage also responds well.[31]

How does ginkgo do all this? Part of the answer probably

lies in the way it improves blood flow. It would help bring in more nutrients through the tiny blood vessels of the inner ear and wash away toxins. Ginkgo also probably has a protective effect on the cells in the brain that are involved in regulating the amount of sound we hear. It may also work directly on the cells of the inner ear themselves.

Impotence

Not often talked about but often dreaded: impotence. It's ruined more than a few people's quality of life. Clinics have been set up around the world to help deal with it; you can see them advertised in places like the sports pages of newspapers. Most cases of impotence are caused by psychological factors. Nonetheless these clinics peddle drugs like Viagra or expensive do-it-yourself injections into the penis. I don't doubt that these are an appropriate treatment in some cases. They're such a lucrative treatment, though, that I'm sure they are overprescribed.

While I was an intern working in an emergency room, I treated a man who had recently been to one of these clinics. He had been under a lot of psychological stress—the number-one cause of impotence—but the clinic did no counseling or anything else to address it. He was also a smoker—another major cause of impotence—but the staff hadn't told him to quit. Instead, they had given him a bunch of needles and drugs to inject himself with—and a bill for two thousand dollars. Unfortunately they had given him too high of a dose, and the injections had nearly destroyed his penis. He had come into the ER in agony as a result. But I digress.

Traditional Chinese physicians have used ginkgo to treat impotence for hundreds of years. Science, too, now agrees that ginkgo looks like a promising treatment for the minority of cases of impotence that are due to arterial disease. In two separate studies in the last decade, patients with impotence, many of whom had not been helped by other drugs, were given ginkgo. About half of them were cured, and many others significantly improved.[32]

Unlike injected drugs, ginkgo doesn't override one's natural reflexes and cause an erection on its own, so there's no danger of damage to the penis, as in the case I described above. Ginkgo just makes erections easier to obtain.

The Tree of Longevity

In traditional Chinese medicine, ginkgo has for centuries been used for the diseases of the elderly and as a longevity tonic. Maybe it is because ginkgo is a very long-lived species, with individual trees living two thousand years or more, that the ancients believed it could confer long life.

The ancients' reasoning actually makes a lot of sense scientifically. We know now that the very same bioflavonoid compounds in ginkgo that protect the trees themselves from oxidative damage, enabling them to withstand radiation and toxins and to live longer, also protect us and help us live longer. The healing forces of nature can heal us, too. It's one of the marvels of interconnectedness within the natural world. We really are much less separate from nature than we often believe.

Just as the Chinese herbalists have also always known, ginkgo is more than a brain booster and a longevity tonic. In the next chapter, we'll explore further ginkgo's amazingly broad range of medicinal powers.

Chapter 5

GINKGO HEALS ASTHMA, ALLERGIES, DIABETES, PMS, AND MORE

Soothing Asthma and Allergies

Legends tell of how Emperor Shen Nong, also known as "the pharmacist sage," devoted his days to the study of nature and its healing forces. Living five thousand years ago, he is said to have first developed the concepts of yin and yang. He was also the first to catalogue hundreds of herbal medicines—all of which he tested on himself. Shen Nong became the patron of Chinese apothecaries and herbalists. Twice a month, on the full and the new moons, they brought offerings to his shrines, and they customarily sold their herbs at discounted prices at those times. Even today his writings retain their authoritative status in traditional Chinese medicine.[1]

It is from his venerated texts that we know that ginkgo has long been used for conditions of the lungs as well as the heart. This tradition has survived to the present day, and practitioners in Chinese clinics still prescribe a tea of ginkgo leaves to treat asthma and bronchitis.

The more Western science examines traditional Chinese medicine, the more it learns about the validity and wisdom of this ancient system of healing. The use of ginkgo tea for asthma is a case in point, because modern research shows that ginkgo extracts really do help heal this common condition.

A group of researchers in the department of pharmacology at the University of London have published studies on the effects of different ginkgolides on asthma and allergies.[2] They've discovered that these compounds powerfully ease the bronchial narrowing caused by exposure to allergens. It seems that ginkgolides act by reducing inflammation around small airways in the lungs. This is a major plus for asthma sufferers, since airway inflammation is probably the most troublesome aspect of the disease.

People with asthma know that in many cases treating the early response to an allergen—the first wheezing you feel when you get a whiff of pollen, for example—is not that difficult. You can often get rid of it with a few puffs of ventolin. That's because the early response is caused by muscle spasm in the walls of the airways, and all you need to do to open up the airways again is to relax those muscles. It's the late response—waking you up at night short of breath, long after the allergen exposure—that tends to be more resistant to treatment. Rather than being due to muscle spasm, the late response is due to the slow accumulation of fluid and inflammatory cells, blocking off the flow of air.

Conventional Western doctors generally recommend treatment with steroids to prevent the late response. In most cases the steroids are inhaled, but when the illness becomes more severe, they are taken in tablet form. Unfortunately even the low doses of steroids delivered by inhalers can cause side effects like oral candida infection, and suppress the body's hormones.

Ginkgo, like steroids, can prevent the late response. But as one randomized, double-blind study demonstrated, it can do so with no side effects whatsoever.[3] It's also effective in exercise-induced asthma.[4] As a bonus, ginkgo is also a good treatment for allergic skin rashes.[5] This, too, sets it apart from conventional medications for asthma.

It's the PAF-blocking capacities of the ginkgolides that give them their power against allergic illnesses. Apart from causing blood clots, PAF is also responsible for promoting inflammation. As it happens, people with allergies are more sensitive to PAF than other people.[6] So the PAF blockers in ginkgo are ideal for helping bring the allergy sufferer's system back into balance.

Even apart from the ginkgolides, at least seven other substances in ginkgo are known to be effective in treating allergies, including the bioflavonoids quercetin, kaempherol, and others.[7] It's almost as if ginkgo were especially designed to treat allergies.

But here's where the relationship between ginkgo and allergies gets really interesting: ginkgo pollen is itself a potent allergen. In areas where the tree is planted in large numbers, as in Southeast Asia, it causes widespread outbreaks of hay fever each spring.[8] Ginkgo fruit is highly allergenic, too. It causes a severe rash in those who handle it, and gastrointestinal upset in those who eat it.[9] So although ginkgo is very good at treating allergies, it's very good at causing them, too.

This peculiar situation reminds me of the concept in homeopathic philosophy known as the Law of Similars. A disease can be cured, say the homeopaths, by a medicine that produces the same symptoms as the disease. So it seems perfectly logical to them that ginkgo, which causes allergies, can also cure allergies.

It's fascinating how many times this Law of Similars is verified in conventional medicine. Almost all the drugs used for cancer chemotherapy, for example, are highly carcinogenic. The drug digoxin, used to treat certain irregularities of heart rhythm, itself causes those exact same irregularities if taken by healthy people. And so on.

Ginkgo's relationship with allergies also seems to bear out an even older saying: *The remedy is created before the disease.*

Protection from Diabetes

Ginkgo has a unique role to play in the treatment of diabetes, too. One thing that makes diabetes so difficult to treat is that it affects so many parts of the body. It's an illness that can start out with inflammation in just a few tiny areas in the pancreas—the islets of Langerhans, which make insulin and other hormones. Over the course of years, it can go on to cause serious damage to the eyes, nerves, kidneys, heart, and all the arteries. The person often ends up needing to take piles of different medications for these various problems. But it's precisely the widespread nature of diabetes that makes ginkgo look so promising in its treatment. As studies show, it can help protect all of those organs from damage.

First, we need to understand what goes wrong with the organs of people with diabetes. When blood sugar levels are high, sugar chemically bonds to proteins all over the body. This turns the proteins into a kind of sludge, most of which gets deposited in the walls of blood vessels. This weakens the blood vessels, making them prone to leak. The cells outside the blood vessels start to starve, since the deposits block the flow of oxygen and nutrients to them. This is why diabetes can cause problems in the heart, the kidney, and the retina of the eye—these tissues all require a lot of oxygen and nutrients.

But because ginkgo improves blood flow in small arteries, it is a good medicine for diabetics. In fact, good hard evidence backs up this reasoning.

In a double-blind, placebo-controlled trial from France, for example, 29 patients with early diabetic retinopathy (retinal damage) were treated with ginkgo extract for six months.[10] The patients on the placebo, as expected, experienced a worsening of their vision due to the continuing sludge buildup in the small blood vessels of the retina. The patients receiving ginkgo, in contrast, had an improvement in their vision. Ginkgo didn't just prevent further damage to their retinas; it actually healed some of the damage that had already been done. It opened up the flow through the sludge-clogged blood vessels, allowing the retina to receive its proper nourishment again.

Ginkgo can do the same thing for the heart, as I discussed in the last chapter. It improves vascular disease of the brain and limbs, which is especially relevant for diabetics, since they suffer disproportionately from these problems. Another recent study suggests that ginkgo may also play a role in the prevention of diabetic neuropathy (nerve damage).[11]

By improving blood flow and oxygen delivery to the whole body, ginkgo is an all-around healer in diabetes. Importantly, unlike some drugs used to treat diabetes and cardiovascular disease, ginkgo extract itself causes no disturbances in blood sugar regulation.[12]

Relief from PMS

Up to 90 percent of women suffer from premenstrual syndrome (PMS), according to some studies. Its symptoms include restlessness, irritability, tension, and fluid retention, all occurring in the second half of the menstrual cycle. Ginkgo has shown some potential in this hard-to-treat illness as well. In 1993 a randomized trial with 165 women found that ginkgo worked significantly better than a placebo for PMS. It was especially good for relieving bloating or congestion, but it also helped with the psychological symptoms.[13]

Ginkgo has also been studied in other, less common conditions related to fluid retention, like acute mountain sickness, and it is quite effective in restoring normal fluid balance to the body.[14] It does so by normalizing the function of leaky capillaries, stopping the buildup of excess fluid in the tissues.

Boosting Immunity and Healing

Researchers have recently discovered that ginkgo extract has powerful effects on the immune system, bringing it back into balance if it's not functioning properly.[15] Ginkgo's potential is high, therefore, for helping many conditions associated with imbalanced immunity—conditions as diverse as psoriasis and organ transplants.

Ginkgo can also speed the healing process itself. At the cellular level healing is about rebuilding and repairing. Proteins and other molecules are assembled carefully and put into place by specialized cells called fibroblasts. A 1997 study showed that ginkgo extracts enhance the development and function of human fibroblasts.[16] When the tissue cultures were treated with ginkgo extract, more collagen and other structural proteins were laid down. In another recent study, ginkgo decreased the breakdown of tissues by bacteria.[17] These effects add up to an increased rate of wound healing.

More Possibilities for Ginkgo

Ginkgo performs such interesting and unique actions on the body that researchers have been inspired to investigate its uses for a wide variety of conditions. Its protective effects against toxins, for example, mean that it could be a useful herb to take along with certain synthetic medications, to lessen their toxic effects on the body.[18]

Ginkgo also shows promise in the treatment of chronic hepatitis—a serious illness, affecting more than a million people in the United States alone. A 1995 study found ginkgo to be effective in preventing and even reversing liver damage in people with chronic hepatitis B infections. This clinical study examined 86 patients, each of whom had a liver biopsy before and then after three months of treatment with ginkgo. After treatment the researchers found that the ongoing process of liver scarring in these patients had actually gone into remission. This preliminary study was not randomized or double-blinded, but its results were so positive that it remains very clinically significant.[19]

As ginkgo's many exciting possibilities have become clear, more and more research groups around the world have begun to study it. But this increased research raises the question: with all ginkgo's beneficial effects, and with European doctors wholeheartedly endorsing it, why do most American doctors know nothing about it? Or for that matter, about any herb? In the next chapter, we'll look at the story behind this bizarre situation.

Because of all these remarkable healing actions, the drug companies have been racing to develop a synthetic, patentable drug that can do what ginkgo can. So far, they haven't even come close.

Chapter 6

WHY MOST DOCTORS KNOW NOTHING ABOUT HERBS

The Unscientific Truth About Conventional American Medicine

Ginkgo is just one of many botanical medicines that science has proven to be effective and safe. A few examples of others: St. John's Wort, ginger, echinacea, milk thistle, ginseng, garlic, hawthorn, and licorice. In European countries like France and Germany, herbs are a major part of mainstream medical care. So what's going on here in the United States? Why do most American doctors ignore herbs? Why do they continue to prescribe toxic synthetic drugs, even when they're no more effective than herbs?

My physician colleagues have given me the same answers time after time: "There isn't enough evidence," or "The studies just aren't good enough." I've discovered, though, that anyone who gives me an answer like that has most likely looked at only two or three studies on herbs at the most. The truth is that most American doctors just don't read the journals that publish research on herbs. Most American doctors know next to nothing about herbs and fall back on the old "there isn't enough evidence" line to dismiss the subject.

I predict that doctors here will eventually change their prescribing habits though—because their patients will demand it. In this Age of Information, news of scientific advances, such as the breakthrough studies on ginkgo, is becoming more and more accessible to all of us. People are already learning about the many safe and effective treatments that alternative medicine offers, and they're demanding them as never before.

But why don't all doctors in the English-speaking world know about ginkgo and other herbs? I think a number of factors in the medical system work against widespread acceptance of herbs. Simple ignorance and prejudice against herbal medications are two big factors. But overshadowing them by far are the financial and political influences that the drug companies exert on the medical profession.

The Reign of the Drug Companies

The goal of the drug companies is basically the same as that of all other companies: to make money. They do a very good job of it. The global market for antidepressants alone, for instance, is estimated to be worth nearly six *billion* dollars annually. But because of extensive legislation, the drugs that these giant multinational companies produce are very expensive to research and develop. As a result, the companies need to get a high return on them to recoup their expenses. The only way the companies can get the high returns that they need is to be able to patent the drugs they produce. That way, they can hold a monopoly on them and charge whatever they like for them, ensuring that they will cover their expenses and make a hefty profit to boot.

Unlike synthetic drugs, herbs are not patentable. Anyone can grow them and sell them, driving down the price and the profit margin. It doesn't make financial sense for drug companies to do research on herbs or market them. Since the overwhelming majority of research on medications is funded by drug companies, nonpatentable medications such as herbs tend to be systematically ignored.

All of this would not be so bad if doctors were not so dependent on the pharmaceutical industry. Most doctors receive most of their information about their own profession from the drug companies, either directly, through advertising, seminars, freebies, and so on, or indirectly, by relying on the recommendations of academic specialists, who are frequently in the employ of drug companies. This information, apart from generally ignoring safer alternatives to synthetic drugs, is often extremely biased or downright misleading. Side effects are often glossed over or ignored.

Most doctors have a fatalistic attitude about side effects anyway. "There are two kinds of drugs," goes the medical saying, "drugs with side effects, and drugs that don't work." Such attitudes are symptomatic of the therapeutic pessimism that pervades conventional medicine. And this saying ignores the fact that some medications cause frequent and severe side effects, while others are virtually free of them.

Patients, understandably, are not so blasé about these matters. Side effects are the most common cause of noncompliance with synthetic medications and therefore are probably the most common cause of treatment failure. Even in scientific studies, for instance, where patients and doctors are more highly motivated than in everyday practice, 21 percent of patients quit taking Ticlid, the synthetic drug most similar to ginkgo, because they couldn't stand the side effects: severe gastrointestinal upset, rashes, and a drop in the white blood cell count, causing impaired immunity.[1] In everyday practice the percentage is probably closer to 30 or 40 percent—but doctors don't really know for sure, because patients often won't admit to giving up the drug, for fear of "letting down" the doctor.

In contrast, because ginkgo is so much better tolerated than synthetic drugs, patients are much less likely to give it up. In a large study of patients taking ginkgo extract, only 1.2 percent of them quit because of side effects.[2]

Why Herbs Are Better

The blame for the medical profession's failure to use herbs like ginkgo does not lie entirely with the drug companies. After all, doctors are the ones who write the prescriptions. The fact is that many doctors are simply prejudiced against herbs. They think herbalists are selling hocus-pocus and fairy tales, more akin to snake oil than medicine. To some extent the alternative health industry has brought this prejudice on itself. Too often it has made claims for its products that are far beyond the scientific truth. Even today it's difficult to separate the hype from the facts in the health food industry.

As a result, though many doctors are curious about herbal medications, a generalized belief prevails in the profession that herbs are only "pretend" drugs, more likely to do harm than good. This prejudice is further supported by the conspicuous absence of information about herbs in the medical education that doctors receive. The only times herbal medications were mentioned in my medical school curriculum were when we were instructed to look out for licorice poisoning as a cause of high blood pressure, and comfrey as a cause of hepatic vein thrombosis. Many conventional medications, we were informed, like aspirin, morphine, quinine, and digoxin, had initially been extracted from herbs, but this process of extraction and refinement of the effective ingredient, we were taught, made the final product far superior. Refinement supposedly provided a purer drug by eliminating the myriad other "useless" compounds found in the original herb. The resultant refined product, then, was said to be (theoretically) more effective, more predictable in its effects, and therefore safer.

That sounds reasonable, and I accepted it as true—until I learned a few basic facts about herbs. The truth is that the standard medical dogma contains some seriously mistaken ideas about herbs, as medical herbalist Dr. Andrew Weil points out in his book *Health and Healing.* "The idea that plants owe their effects to single compounds is simply untrue," he writes. "Drug plants are always complex mixtures of chemicals, all of which contribute to the effect of the whole." They do usually contain one ingredient in a higher concentration than the others, he explains, but the variety of other similar compounds in the plant work synergistically with it to produce an overall effect greater than that which could be produced by any one ingredient alone.[3]

Opium, as an example, contains not only morphine but also a variety of other opioids, like papaverine and codeine, each with a slightly different action in the body. Papaverine, for instance, is a muscle relaxant and thereby provides pain relief through a mechanism different from morphine's, hence supplementing its effects. Similarly, scientists have been unable to locate any single substance in ginkgo that alone accounts for all of its actions. As I've discussed in previous chapters, it contains a number of different substances that are the effective ingredients, and they enhance one anothers' actions. Extracts of the whole leaf therefore have properties far beyond those of any one of its ingredients.

Because herbs produce a variety of synergistic healing effects, the overall dose of an herbal medication can be smaller, and less concentrated, than that of a synthetic drug. Toxicity is therefore much less likely to occur. Interestingly, even conventional pharmacologists (doctors who study the use of drugs) sometimes recommend that patients in whom side effects from a single drug are a problem use a variety of different drugs together in low doses. But this was nature's answer all along. Nature packages lots of different healing ingredients together in low doses in one herb.

Another reason herbs are less toxic is that their active ingredients are less concentrated than refined drugs and are often less soluble, so they are more slowly absorbed. This produces steadier, lower concentrations of medicine in the system—a sort of built-in safety mechanism. Synthetic drugs, by contrast, are plagued by problems of toxicity due to their rapid absorption. They reach high peak levels in the bloodstream, then rapidly fall again, making the correct dose of a drug difficult to achieve. The levels seesaw back and forth between the therapeutic range and the toxic range. Recently many conventional drugs have become available in "sustained release" forms, which are absorbed more slowly, with fewer toxic peak levels. But again, this was nature's answer all along.

Thus herbal medications, contrary to the dogma with which doctors are presented during their medical education, are generally much safer, and often as effective as refined drugs. Ginkgo is a case in point.

The Future of Ginkgo

Ginkgo, having become one of the most frequently prescribed medications of any type, has taken the drug market in Europe by storm. Because it's nonpatentable, no one drug company can hold a monopoly on it, so its price will always be competitive. As a result, the big synthetic drug companies will probably never offer it for sale. But you can bet they're keeping a very close eye on ginkgo. It will undoubtedly take a big bite out of their American profits from drugs like Cognex, Aricept, and Ticlid—synthetic drugs that have some effects similar to ginkgo.

What the drug companies would like to do is go to their chemistry labs and develop a synthetic version of ginkgo. They would then take out a patent on it and spend lots of money on research and marketing, trying to convince doctors that it was better than the original form of ginkgo. But they probably won't be able to do it, because natural ginkgolides are extremely difficult to synthesize. They are "cage" molecules, meaning they are shaped like small, three-dimensional cages, and so far no one has developed a method for replicating them artificially.

The closest the companies have come to a synthetic version of ginkgo is possibly the drug Ticlid, which I mentioned in previous chapters. It's not a cage molecule like the ginkgolides, but it inhibits platelet-activating factor (PAF) just as they do. It's prescribed to decrease the stickiness of platelets and thin the blood. Compared with ginkgo, however, it has a huge number of side effects, and it's very expensive. It has only a small fraction of the other beneficial effects that ginkgo has. So unless the drug companies can discover some way to synthesize ginkgolides, ginkgo may just remain an unbeatable adversary for them.

Other vested interests in the medical establishment may

try to oppose ginkgo, too. Health insurance associations, for instance, may try to save money by discouraging doctors from prescribing it. This actually happened in Germany about ten years ago. Throughout the 1980s ginkgo prescriptions had been costing the German health insurance companies millions of Deutschmarks each year, and the number being written had been climbing steadily. If the insurance companies could persuade doctors to stop prescribing it, they would save all this money. So in 1989 a German health insurance association sent out negative information about ginkgo to doctors.[4] The manufacturers of ginkgo took legal action against the insurance association, stating that the information was misinterpreted and false. The court granted an injunction against the insurance association, but the association appealed it, and the appeal was then upheld on the basis of freedom of expression. The court explicitly stated that no conclusion had been reached with regard to the effectiveness of ginkgo or otherwise.[5]

Clearly, not much of a dent was made in ginkgo's popularity by this attack—the number of prescriptions continued to rise steadily. The incident illustrates well, though, the kind of opposition ginkgo might face in this country. HMOs here are always interested in cost cutting and will probably try to avoid putting ginkgo on their formularies. On the other hand, its low cost could also mean it will be included.

Fortunately we all have access to ginkgo ourselves. Herbal medications are on sale everywhere, and even though the FDA may be trying to restrict our access to them, the situation isn't likely to change in the near future.

By now, since you have access to it, you're probably wondering whether ginkgo is right for you. In the next chapter, you'll find some more important points to consider in making that decision.

Chapter 7

USING GINKGO SAFELY

So far you've read about how ginkgo has helped other people. Maybe you're wondering if it's right for you. In this chapter we'll look at how to make that decision, then go over some basic points for using ginkgo safely.

Proper Diagnosis: An Essential

Point number one: if you're ill, take ginkgo only with the cooperation of your doctor. The care of a doctor is vital not only for diagnosis and prescribing but for monitoring the effects of treatment. For your own sake, your doctor should be involved with your decision to use ginkgo, in the unlikely event that anything untoward does happen, like an unusual side effect. And as mentioned previously, ginkgo is not for everybody—you may need a different approach to treatment.

How can you make sure that you're being prescribed the best treatment for your particular condition? Talk to your doctor. Tell them that you've read about ginkgo and would like to try it. If they haven't caught up with the research on it, show them this book, or give them a photocopy of appendix 4. It provides references for recent journal articles that are easily available and a good starting point for learning about ginkgo. Once your doctors know about ginkgo, they will probably be willing to prescribe it. If they're not, ask why. Don't assume they're closed-minded. They may have good reasons for not wanting to prescribe it for you. It's not suitable for everyone. For example, if you are taking aspirin regularly, I wouldn't recommend that you mix ginkgo with it.

In spite of my criticisms of doctors in the last chapter, I have to say that most doctors I know are very open-minded, reasonable people. If something has been demonstrated to work in proper scientific trials, they will generally accept it. After all, they do want the best for their patients. With ginkgo's remarkable track record, it's really just a matter of time before doctors will start prescribing it.

When You Should Not Use Ginkgo

There are a few situations where ginkgo should not be used, and it's important for you to know about them.

Pregnant women should not take ginkgo. Any medicine carries a risk of birth defects. True, none have been reported with ginkgo, but studies haven't been done on this issue yet. So you need to play it safe. Likewise, if you're a woman in your childbearing years and there is any chance you might become pregnant, you should not use this herb. Nursing women and children under 12 should not use ginkgo. No studies have been done on the use of this herb in babies or young children. They have different metabolisms from adults, and until we know more, it should not be given to them.

People who have disorders of blood clotting, like hemophilia, or a known vitamin K deficiency, should not use ginkgo. They may be at increased risk of bleeding. Likewise, people using drugs that affect blood clotting should avoid ginkgo (see page 86).

People who have an allergy to ginkgo preparations should obviously not take it either. If you're prone to migraines, you should probably start with a lower dose of ginkgo. (See chapter 10 for further details.)

Ginkgo seems to be quite safe for people with liver or kidney disease. It may even be therapeutic for them, as we saw in chapter 5. Unlike many synthetic medications ginkgo doesn't interfere with the liver's detoxification system, which is good news for everyone taking it.[1] If you do have a disease of the liver or kidneys, however, you should receive ginkgo, or any medication for that matter, only under close medical supervision. The liver and kidneys are the body's disposal system, and if they're not working, medicines can easily build up in the body and reach toxic levels.

Drugs That Interact with Ginkgo

Other medications can potentially cause problems if mixed with ginkgo, and I recommend that they should not be taken with it. Aspirin is one of them. Like ginkgo, aspirin thins the blood, protecting against abnormal clotting. But it can also cause problems with bleeding. In a recent case report in the *New England Journal of Medicine,* a man who had been taking aspirin regularly for years experienced spontaneous bleeding in his eye a week after he started taking ginkgo.[2] It was probably the combined effects of the aspirin and the ginkgo that did it.

This same effect might also foreseeably occur with certain pain-relieving medications, such as the nonsteroidal anti-inflammatory drugs (NSAIDs), including Motrin, Indocin, and Voltaren, among others. (See pages 87–88.) I would avoid these as well.

Another drug that might increase the risk of bleeding if mixed with ginkgo is the synthetic PAF-inhibitor Ticlid. The same goes for Persantine, which also affects platelets.

Natural alternatives to the synthetic blood thinners may be safer. White willow bark, the original source of aspirin, has been used in traditional Chinese medicine for at least 2,500 years. It causes fewer problems with stomach upset than aspirin does, and it's said to result in a lower risk of bleeding. Similarly, the Chinese wood ear mushroom (also called tree ear or ear fungus) can effectively thin the blood. It's a common ingredient in Chinese stir-fries, is available in Chinese grocery stores, and is also quite safe.

The humble garlic clove is another, better known natural way to thin your blood. Raw onions have a similar action. Fish oils and flax oil also have gentle blood-thinning capabilities.

Vitamin E is another natural blood thinner, as well as a powerful antioxidant and anti-aging medicine. It's not so much the vitamin E itself that thins the blood as a metabolite called vitamin E-quinone. With high doses of vitamin E, enough of this metabolite can accumulate to cause problems in some individuals. You can decrease the amount of vitamin E-quinone that is formed in your body if you take vitamin C along with the E. Nevertheless, if you have a disorder of blood clotting or are on drugs that interfere with blood clotting, I would not use vitamin E supplements.

Use Caution When Taking Ginkgo with These Drugs

- Aspirin: including Ecotrin, Acuprin, Norgesic, Fiorinal, Excedrin, and other aspirin products.
- NSAIDs: including Aleve, Anaprox, and Naprosyn (all brand names of naproxen), Cataflam and Voltaren (types of diclofenac), Motrin and Advil (ibuprofen), Feldene (piroxicam), Indocin (indomethacin), Orudis (ketoprofen), and others

- Ticlid (ticlopidine)
- Plavix (clopidogrel)
- Persantine (dipyridamole)
- Heparin, Fragmin, Lovenox
- Coumadin (warfarin)

The above guidelines are very conservative, and you will not find them published anywhere else. In fact, the 1994 German government's official monograph on ginkgo states that it has no known interactions with other medications, no known restrictions for pregnancy or lactation, and only one contraindication to its use: allergy to ginkgo preparations.[3] Still, if you have any of those conditions, or are on any of those medications, I advise you not to take ginkgo. You do not want to be the first one to have a bad reaction to it. Play it safe.

Why Medication Isn't Enough

So far we've looked at the question of how to get the best medication for your particular circumstances. But for any condition medication is really only one part of a good overall treatment plan. Used alone, it's inadequate. That goes for ginkgo, too.

If you're thinking about using ginkgo for its nootropic effect, for instance, you should be aware that lifestyle modifications may be even more effective in increasing your brain power. Regular exercise increases the blood flow to the brain and improves the balance of neurotransmitters involved in memory, concentration, and alertness. Switching over to a high-complex-carbohydrate, low-sugar-and-fat diet can improve your ability to think clearly, too. That means a mainly vegetarian diet, low in sugar. Add more fish to your diet, too. It contains omega-3 fatty acids, which are very brain friendly. I'd also invest in a good-quality multivitamin and mineral preparation. If you're using sleeping tablets, sedatives, recreational drugs, or more than a small amount of alcohol, stopping these will obviously help as well.

Exercising your brain is important, too. A recent study in the journal *Life Sciences* demonstrated conclusively that ginkgo has complementary and synergistic effects with memory training.[4] One of the best ways to exercise your memory is to learn a new language.

If you're using ginkgo for life extension, the above lifestyle factors also apply to you. But probably the most effective way to extend your life span is simply to eat less. Eating a low-calorie diet slows your basal metabolic rate, the clock for the aging process. This does not mean dieting to lose weight, but rather balanced, healthy eating.

If you're considering giving ginkgo to a family member with dementia, you need to be aware of the many other options that alternative medicine offers. Nutritional therapy is one of the basics. A broad range of antioxidants, including selenium and vitamins E and C, should supplement a diet rich in fish and colorful fruits and vegetables like dark grapes, blueberries, broccoli, and red peppers. Dark-colored fruits and vegetables are especially full of healthy bioflavonoids.

Drinking a glass of dark grape juice daily is one easy way to increase your bioflavonoid intake. I'd add flax oil or evening primrose oil supplements, too, to ensure an adequate intake of essential fatty acids. Avoiding synthetic oils and fried foods is important. Making these dietary changes will help quench the chronic, low-grade inflammation in the brain that is one of the root causes of Alzheimer's. Chelation therapy is cited by many doctors as an effective treatment for Alzheimer's as well. Regular exercise and mental stimulation are crucial.

As you can see from these examples, ginkgo should just be one part of the story. A holistic approach, involving all aspects of a person's life, is the most effective way to treat any condition. Holistic medicine is about more than just biochemistry, and it uses more than just medication. It takes into account all of the other aspects of a person's life and treats them as a whole being—mind, body, and spirit together.

Holistic medical practitioners—M.D.'s, D.O.'s, and others—are qualified in conventional medicine, but they choose to work within this larger framework of understanding human beings. When it comes to diagnosis and treatment, they consider much more than symptoms alone. They look carefully at all parts of the person's world, in order to understand what the symptoms mean in the context of that person's life. They consider the person's diet, exercise, relaxation, and work habits, for instance. Many of the things going in the person's social, cultural, mental, and spiritual life, they understand, have a great influence on how they are feeling. The person's relationships with their family, for example, are very important. So are their goals in life, and their beliefs, and whether they're living the kind of life they really want.

In other words, holistic doctors take into account the many important ways that a person's mind and spirit affect their body, and vice versa. To treat people on all these levels, they employ a variety of techniques, including nutritional medicine, herbalism, acupuncture, counseling, meditation, homeopathy, physical manipulation, and many other alternative therapies, in addition to the tools of conventional medicine. Most holistic doctors believe that the person's own innate healing mechanisms should be supported and enhanced rather than overridden with drugs and surgery. If conventional medication or surgery is really necessary, though, they will use them. In short, they offer the only truly comprehensive medical care available.

To locate a medical doctor in your area who practices according to the principles of holistic medicine, refer to appendix 3. I've found in my own work that when patients are treated holistically, and the underlying causes of their illness dealt with, they can blossom as never before in their lives. In many cases, it's almost as though their illness were a kind of messenger to them, telling them that something in their life needed to be transformed—either within them, or in their lifestyle, or both.

Ginkgo remains a superb medication, and an important part of the overall treatment plan for many patients. It may be for you, too. In the chapters to come, we'll discuss the practical issues of how to buy and use ginkgo.

Chapter 8

HOW TO BUY GINKGO

Where to Buy It

Most health food stores carry ginkgo. If it's not in stock, the proprietor will usually be happy to order it for you. With the general public's increasing appreciation of the value of herbal medications, ginkgo has become available in many grocery stores, discount stores, and pharmacies. Many naturopaths and other natural healers can supply ginkgo, so if you have no nearby retail supplier, you could try looking these practitioners up in your Yellow Pages.

If these options aren't convenient for you, you can order ginkgo through the mail, or over the phone, or by fax, or through the Internet, from many companies. Appendix 1 lists some of these suppliers and how to contact them.

Ginkgo is sold in a number of forms, and deciding which one is right for your needs can be confusing. This section provides a summary of the reasons you might want to pick one form over the others.

The 50:1 Standardized Extract

The form in which you'll most commonly find ginkgo being sold is the 50:1 standardized extract. The "50:1" part means that 50 pounds of leaves were used to make one pound of the finished extract. The "standardized" part means that the manufacturers ensured that a particular percentage of the active ingredients were present in each batch. You can be fairly well assured that a standardized extract is going to have a uniform, predictable effect.

The standardized extract is the most highly processed form of ginkgo you can buy. Many separate steps go into its production. After the leaves are ground up and soaked in the extracting fluid (also called the menstruum), the inactive ingredients, like cellulose, are strained out. The extracting fluid is then mostly removed, leaving a concentrated solution. This solution is then adjusted to achieve the desired concentration of particular ingredients. The whole process takes two weeks and involves twenty-seven separate steps.

The percentages of particular ingredients that the extract contains are written on the label of most ginkgo products. The usual percentages are:

- From 22 to 27 percent (usually 24 percent) *ginkgo flavonglycosides* (also called bioflavonoids or flavonoids). This includes the antioxidant substances *quercetin* and *kaempferol,* discussed in chapter 5.

- From 5 to 7 percent *terpene lactones,* which include the neuroprotective PAF-inhibiting ginkgolides A, B, and C and bilobalide. Some preparations list the percentages of each of these separately. For instance, they might have these percentages: ginkgolide A, 1.2 percent; ginkgolide B, 0.8 percent; ginkgolide C, 1.0 percent; bilobalide, 2.8 percent.

- Less than 5 parts per million of *ginkgolic* or *anacardic acids,* the allergy-producing compounds discussed in chapter 10.

These percentages are the ones that were found to be optimum, through a process of trial and error, back in the 1960s, by German doctor and herbal manufacturer Willmar Schwabe. They were specified by the German government in 1994 for the composition of ginkgo extract. Almost all of the research on ginkgo has used 50:1 extracts that have met these specifications.

For most applications this form of ginkgo is probably the best to use. If you have an illness for which ginkgo extract has been proven to work, you'll get the most predictable results from it. In essence, you'll be repeating the conditions in the studies the most closely.

Can Standardized Extracts Heal a Sick Science?

Some herbalists criticize the use of standardized extracts, pointing out that for thousands of years healers have used simpler preparations, like tea made from dried leaves. Standardized extracts have been around for only a few decades. So it's really the simpler preparations that have the longer track record for safety. Moreover, the process of standardization, say traditional herbalists, also disrupts the balance of compounds found naturally in the leaves. Even the manufacturers of standardized extracts will admit that it does.

Because the standardized extract is so concentrated, for example, manufacturers have to tinker with the levels of one group of ingredients to avoid adverse reactions. They need to ensure that the extract has below five parts per million of ginkgolic acids. When concentrated, these allergy-producing acids can become a real problem, causing inflammation of the stomach lining and intestines. But in the unprocessed ginkgo leaf, ginkgolic acids are present in such low doses that they rarely cause adverse effects. So processing the leaf overrides its built-in safety.

Some skeptics have even claimed that the real reason ginkgo was concentrated in the first place was simply so herb manufacturers could make more money. The herb manufacturers, especially the Schwabe company, funded most of the research on ginkgo extracts. So naturally they made sure that the studies were performed on their own standardized products rather than unprocessed leaves. Anyone who wanted to prescribe ginkgo would have to prescribe a Schwabe product if they wanted to be scientifically based. People who wanted to use the plain, unprocessed leaf form would not have a scientific leg to stand on.

Advocates of standardized extracts answer this criticism by pointing out that the plain leaf form is not strong enough to have much of a medicinal effect. You need to take so much of it, they say, that it becomes too difficult to manage. Capsules are more convenient. Furthermore, it would be difficult to do placebo-controlled studies on the traditional form of taking ginkgo, ginkgo tea, since the patients would clearly see and taste the difference between real ginkgo tea and the placebo tea.

I can see both sides of the argument. More deeply, some fundamental issues about the nature of herbs, and even the universe, are being debated here. One of these issues concerns the question of whether things in the world have a divine purpose. Many herbalists believe that medicinal herbs were specifically placed on earth by divine grace. This was, in fact, a basic tenet of herbalism before the modern era. If you believe it, then you are bound to question any kind of artificial alterations made to herbs. It would be interfering with the divine order of things.

A possible reply to this argument would be that human beings were also given intelligence by divine grace— intelligence to use the things they found in the world in the most effective way possible. Modifying herbs might not be contrary to the divine plan after all—on the contrary, it might be what was intended.

Another issue underlying this debate is the relationship between herbalism and conventional medicine. When herbs are broken down, analyzed, standardized, and studied in clinical trials, the people doing it are often trying to bridge the gap between the two approaches to healing. But should herbalists strive to be part of conventional medicine? Should they try to be scientific at all? In the eyes of many people in the alternative medicine scene, conventional medicine is a corrupt, misguided system that hurts patients more than it heals them. At its core lies a fundamental mistake—a science based on the separation of mind and body. This philosophy of Cartesian dualism has alienated us all from the earth, say some opponents of conventional science, and led to widespread destruction of the environment and native cultures. Why try to be like that?

A possible reply would be that bringing herbs into the realm of conventional medicine would itself be a kind of healing. The main sickness of conventional medicine is that it denies that we are one with the earth. The introduction of herbs could help heal this false belief. Conventional doctors and their patients might once again appreciate the earth's own medicines. We would be spurred on to help preserve nature rather than destroy it. For example, we might try harder to halt the destruction of the South American and Asian rain forests if we could better appreciate the priceless medicinal plant species in them that are becoming extinct every day.

These are the reasons I believe bringing herbal medicines into the realm of conventional medicine is a very good thing, both for humans and for the earth. If it takes standardization to achieve it, then so be it.

Nonstandardized Extracts

Ginkgo is sometimes sold in the form of nonstandardized extracts. They can come either in capsules or as a liquid extract. The capsule form is produced very much like the standardized extract, except that the percentages of the ingredients are not adjusted. The liquid extracts are made by soaking ground-up leaves in alcohol or glycerine, allowing the oily active ingredients to dissolve out into the liquid. The inactive residue of the leaves is then strained out. (Alcohol-based extracts are also known as tinctures.) The extracts are usually sold in small brown glass bottles, with a medicine dropper that screws into the top. The dark glass protects against light-induced degradation. It's best to store them in the refrigerator, to protect against heat-induced degradation, too.

Most labels also contain the words "Fresh herb: Menstruum ratio 1:1.5," or "Fresh herb strength 1:1," or something similar. This bit of herbal technicalese is basically a statement about how strong the extract is. The ratio indicates the proportion of ground-up leaves to alcohol or glycerine in the extract. The potencies of nonstandardized extracts vary quite a lot between different products, even between different batches of the same product.

Nonstandardized extracts are usually cheaper than standardized ones. An advantage of the alcohol-based liquid extract is that alcohol is a very good carrier of some of the less water-soluble compounds in the leaves, and it may deliver them to the body more rapidly and more completely than other ginkgo preparations. It's said that if you take the alcohol-based extract on an empty stomach, you can get an onset of a nootropic effect within 30 seconds.

The main drawback of less concentrated extracts is that they are probably less effective. The research here is limited, but one study comparing a concentrated ginkgo extract with an unconcentrated one in the treatment of heart disease found that while both were effective, the concentrated extract worked better for moderate to severe disease.[1] You may be able to overcome this problem by simply taking more of the extract, but then you would run the risk of ingesting enough ginkgolic acids to irritate your stomach. You would also lose the cost advantage. Then again, if you made your own extract, which is easy to do, cost wouldn't be a factor. (See chapter 11 for details.)

Considering all these points, nonstandardized extracts would be reasonable to use if you don't have a serious illness. In that case, you don't require the degree of therapeutic certainty that standardized extracts offer.

Unprocessed Ginkgo Leaves

The most traditional and least expensive form of ginkgo is unprocessed leaves. No scientific studies support its use, but countless herbalists since prehistoric times approve. You can buy plain ginkgo leaves in two different forms: capsules filled with freeze-dried, ground-up leaves and, in a few health food stores and herbal shops, whole dried leaves. You can, of course, pick the leaves yourself as well.

The problem with raw, dried herbs is that exposure to air and light causes their active ingredients to break down. As a result, their potency is not very reliable. Picking the leaves yourself, or using freeze-dried leaves, is one way of getting around this problem.

As with nonstandardized extracts, unprocessed ginkgo leaves are a fair consideration if you don't have a serious illness.

Is Organic Better?

Yes, it really is. Organically grown herbs are hardier and contain higher concentrations of nutrients and active ingredients. And of course, organic herbs are not covered with synthetic poisons that will end up in your body. There is really no justification for ginkgo to be grown any way other than organically. It is so resistant to pests that it never needs spraying, and since it can grow (albeit slowly) in fairly poor soils, it shouldn't need refined fertilizers.

Some brands of extract are certified to be organic. Certification is important because it provides a system of verification of organic status. Otherwise any grower could claim to be organic while actually spraying pesticides all they want. To be certified as organic, farms have to pass strict inspections on a regular basis.

What Does Wildcrafted *Mean?*

Several brands of extract state on the label that their ginkgo is *wildcrafted*. This means that the trees are allowed to grow wild rather than being cultivated or tended. In other words, wildcrafted ginkgos are not grown on plantations, unlike the majority of commercially raised ginkgos today.

How Much Does It Cost?

Shop around—prices for standardized extracts vary enormously. If you're taking a dose of 120 mg a day (one of the more common doses used in studies, but see chapter 9 on working out your dose), your monthly cost can range from around eight to thirty or more U.S. dollars. Mixtures of ginkgo with other herbs or vitamins tend to have higher prices.

Are Mixtures of Herbs Better?

Ginkgo is sometimes sold in mixtures with other herbs. Master herbalists often use mixtures rather than single herbs to treat their patients, relying on their years of experience to judge the correct herbs and the correct amounts for the recipe.

In general, unless a mixture has been prescribed for you by an herbalist who knows what they're doing, I wouldn't use them. First, if you have an adverse reaction to the mixture, it will be impossible to know which of the herbs in it was responsible. Second, using herbs one at a time is the only way to gauge their individual effectiveness for you. And third, it's important for consumers to know all there is to know about the medicines they're taking. Some mixtures contain so many herbs that it's difficult even for professional herbalists to know all about them and about their possible interactions with each other. Basically, mixtures of herbs make things unnecessarily complicated.

Chapter 9

HOW TO USE GINKGO

In this chapter you'll get the basic, nuts-and-bolts information that will enable you to take ginkgo safely and effectively. You'll learn about how much to take and how often. And just as important, you'll learn how long a period to use it for.

How Much Should I Take?

The dose of the standardized extract that you'll need depends on what condition you have. As a generalization, it's considered that higher doses are needed to treat brain disorders, and lower doses are adequate for disorders of the rest of the body.

The recommendations of the German federal health commission reflect this distinction.[1] For the treatment of brain disorders due to poor circulation, it recommends 120 to 240 mg of extract daily, divided into two or three doses. For disorders of the rest of the body, like leg claudication and inner-ear problems, it recommends 120 to 160 mg daily.

As for Alzheimer's, studies have also shown that 120 to 240 mg is effective. Most of the studies on age-associated memory impairment, on the other hand, have shown good effects with just 120 mg daily. If you're using ginkgo mainly for its longevity-enhancing effects, I would recommend 120 mg as well.

No one has yet proved that higher doses are more effective in the long term than lower ones. I therefore recommend starting at the lower end of the dose ranges and increasing the dose only if, after six weeks, the effects are insufficient. To keep tabs on how effective ginkgo is for you, try keeping a daily diary of your target symptoms. For instance, if you're using ginkgo to treat tinnitus, rate the severity of the ringing on a scale of zero to ten each evening, where zero is no ringing and ten is the worst imaginable ringing. Write the number in your diary or on your calendar. Also note when you started taking a particular dose. That way you'll have a record you can use for comparing the effects of different doses.

If you're a healthy person using ginkgo solely for its nootropic (mind-enhancing) effects, there is less data to guide your choice of a dose. Most of the tests have used single doses, which, as I stated earlier, are probably less effective than treatment for a period of several weeks. The two French studies of short-term memory enhancement in young people used a single dose of 600 mg.[2] Lower doses were not effective. I would not recommend you take 600 mg regularly; I believe it's too high for most people. Granted, I have heard of a person who has taken 1000 mg daily for over a year without any side effects.

One EEG study on healthy young people found that a single dose of just 80 mg produced maximum benefits.[3] Increasing the dose beyond that did not increase the effects. In other words, the best nootropic dose is not at all clear. Individual variation probably ranges widely, from 80 mg up to 600 mg. It's also likely that each person has a ceiling dose of ginkgo, beyond which no further benefits can be obtained. As a general rule, I would always start out on the low end to determine a medication's effects.

To be extra safe, if you plan to use ginkgo in a single dose to boost your memory, such as before an exam, you should take a test dose a day or two prior to the exam. It will help you determine whether you are particularly sensitive to it. You don't want to discover during the exam that you're one of the few people who experience side effects like restlessness from ginkgo.

If you're using nonstandardized extracts, be aware that different products will have different potencies. Only the manufacturer will be able to advise you on the correct dose. Follow the instructions on the label.

How Often Should I Take It?

Three doses per day is what the studies have generally used. Two doses are also okay, according to the German federal commission. Ginkgo definitely needs to be taken more than once a day, since most of its active ingredients are excreted within a few hours.

For the technically minded, the term that describes how long a substance stays in the body is the *elimination half-life*. One half-life is the length of time that it takes to clear half of the dose of the substance out of the body. The half-life of ginkgolide A is 4.5 hours.[4] Ginkgolide B's half-life is around 11 hours, and bilobalide's is around 3 hours.[5] The antioxidant bioflavonoids get cleared out fairly quickly, in 2 to 4 hours.[6]

Can I Overdose on Ginkgo?

Because ginkgo is so nontoxic, it would be extremely difficult, probably impossible, to injure yourself by overdosing on it. Unfortunately animal researchers have gone ahead anyway and done tests on mice to determine the lethal dose. It is too high to be relevant—you simply couldn't swallow enough ginkgo pills to kill yourself. Chalk up another no-brainer to animal testing.

Do I Take It with Meals, or on an Empty Stomach?

Take it with meals. One of the main reasons so many people experience nausea and stomach upset as a side effect of medicines and vitamins is that they take them on an empty stomach. That exposes the stomach lining to high concentrations of the stuff they're taking, and so it gets irritated. A few medications do really need to be taken on an empty stomach, because they get inactivated by food. Ginkgo isn't one of them, though.[7]

It's also easier to remember to take your medicine when you have it with each meal.

How to Make Ginkgo Tea

Tea is made using the dried leaves of ginkgo. Here is how it is done: Add one or two teaspoons of the dried leaf to a cup of boiling water in a small saucepan and let it simmer, covered, for five minutes. Drink two or three of these cups per day, sweetened with honey if you wish. It's helpful to purchase a small teapot with a two- or three-cup capacity, such as the Chinese use to serve green tea. They are available for a few dollars at Chinese food stores around the world. With such a teapot you need make only one batch per day.

Ginkgo is also available commercially in teabags, which are standardized, containing the same dose as standardized capsules. See appendix 2 for suppliers.

How Long Does It Take to Work?

After you swallow a capsule of ginkgo, the active ingredients reach their peak levels in your bloodstream in one or two hours.[8] Studies have shown a significant onset of a nootropic effect in only one hour.[9] The alcohol-based extract starts working even more rapidly, since the alcohol enables the ingredients to be absorbed directly through the walls of your stomach. Some people claim to feel noticeable effects within thirty seconds when they take it on an empty stomach.

The research data is clear, though, that the full effects of ginkgo take two to four weeks to be produced.[10] If you're using the unprocessed leaf form, it can take even longer—from one to nine months.[11]

Keep a Ginkgo Log

Keeping a log is one way to see objectively how ginkgo is working for you. For this exercise, you will need a watch with a timer function, about a dozen index cards, scrap paper, and a logbook or calendar in which to record the results.

First, write a random series of twelve numbers on each card. For example, you could write: 4 9 7 2 5 8 3 0 1 1 4 6. Write a different series of numbers on each card.

Now set the timer on your watch for ten seconds. Turn the cards over, shuffle them, and choose one at random. As you press the start button on the timer, turn the card over. Memorize the series of numbers on the card. When the timer goes off, turn the card back over to the blank side. On the scrap paper write down as many of the numbers as you can, in the correct order. Then check your results. Repeat the exercise with a second card.

The average person will get about seven of the numbers on each card in a row correct and in the right order. Add up the number of consecutive numbers on each card that you got right. For example, if you got six correct on one card and eight on the other card, your score is fourteen. Record your score in your logbook.

Ideally, you should do this exercise before you start taking ginkgo, then every two weeks for twelve weeks or so. It's a very crude test for short-term memory, but it's one way to gauge ginkgo's effects for you.

How Long Should I Take It For?

Make sure you give ginkgo enough time to work fully. An adequate trial should consist of at least six weeks of a full dose. The German federal commission recommends that ginkgo be tried for at least eight weeks in the case of a brain disorder. In the 1997 *JAMA* study of dementia, the patients actually continued to improve on one of the measurement scales for the entire fifty-two weeks.[12] So some benefits of ginkgo become apparent only after a considerable period of time.

For intermittent claudication, you should take ginkgo for at least six weeks. In the case of inner-ear disorders like tinnitus, though, the trial does not need to be as long. If it's not decreasing the ringing in your ears after six weeks, it's probably not working for you.[13]

Assuming ginkgo works for you, and you've had no side effects, should you keep taking it indefinitely? There isn't a definite answer to this question yet. One reason is that at the present time no long-term studies have told us if any side effects show up after prolonged treatment. It's true that ginkgo has been used safely for thousands of years and that many people around the world today have been using it for decades with no problems. Chances are that ginkgo is far safer for long-term use than almost any other medication.

If you're taking ginkgo to treat an illness and have no side effects from it, you can probably keep taking it indefinitely. If you have no illness but are taking it for its longevity-enhancing, cancer-preventing, or nootropic effects, you might consider taking intermittent "drug holidays." You could skip taking it for one month in every six, for instance. You'll save money, and you'll allow your body to come back to its own natural chemistry again.

As I discussed in chapter 4, ginkgo's effects as an antioxidant appear to persist for many months after it is discontinued. So even when you take a drug holiday, you'll still have some of the benefits.

When you discontinue it, do so gradually, cutting down the dose bit by bit over a period of a week or so. Of course, if you're discontinuing it because of a side effect, you can do so immediately, without tapering it off. You're very unlikely to need to do this, though, since the side effects are so rare. In the next chapter we'll take a closer look at what side effects can occur, what causes them, and what you can do to avoid them.

Chapter 10

THE SIDE EFFECTS—AND HOW TO AVOID THEM

Is it safe? That's the first question to ask whenever you are considering a new medication. It's an even more important question than *Is it effective?* because if it's not safe, it doesn't really matter how effective it is—you wouldn't want to use it anyway.

With ginkgo, the answer to that question is the kind you want to hear: *it's very safe*. Side effects are remarkably rare, and even when they do occur, they are almost always mild. In fact, studies have found that ginkgo's side effects are no different from those in patients treated with a placebo.

Still, you need to be aware of the side effects that have been reported. I'm a firm believer in the principle that people should know all that there is to know about the products they buy and use, especially medications. It's bad enough to experience side effects, but it's worse when you haven't been informed about what to expect. There's also another good reason doctors should talk about side effects—many of them are preventable with a few commonsense measures.

The commonest side effects of ginkgo are stomach and intestinal symptoms, headaches, and allergic skin reactions. I'll discuss them shortly and the steps you can take to deal with them. I'll also discuss a number of less common side effects, including bleeding. But first I want to make this point clear: if any side effect occurs when you're taking ginkgo, no matter what it is, tell your doctor about it as soon as possible. It's very important that they know about it, even if it doesn't seem important to you. Thousands of years of use, and new scientific studies too, have proved ginkgo to be quite safe—but everyone is unique in their biochemistry. When it comes to medications, we always need to be alert.

Side Effect 1: Stomach and Intestinal Symptoms

These symptoms include nausea (feeling like you want to vomit), abdominal pains, loss of appetite, and diarrhea. In a study of 2,855 patients taking ginkgo extract, 3.7 percent of them reported these symptoms.[1] All of them found that stopping the medication gave them complete relief. These symptoms also occur in patients taking a placebo and in people on no medication, so the medication may not have been responsible. Since the symptoms resolved on stopping the medication, though, it's likely that the extract really was responsible in at least some of these cases.

Why does ginkgo cause stomach upset? We don't know for

certain, but it may have something to do with its effects on PAF, as described in chapters 5 and 6. Ticlopidine, a synthetic drug that also acts on PAF, also causes such upsets but in much higher proportions—in 30 to 40 percent of people taking it.[2] As I explained in chapter 6, the fact that ticlopidine is a synthetic drug probably explains why it's so much more toxic than ginkgo. In general, the more refined the substance, the less well the body can handle it. Similarly, users of high doses of the more concentrated extracts of ginkgo are also more likely to experience these problems.

Ginkgo also contains some known allergens, which can also cause stomach upset, as I'll discuss on page 116.

PREVENTING STOMACH UPSETS

There are ten simple things that you can do to prevent stomach and intestinal symptoms from ginkgo, or to decrease them if you have them:

1. Take your ginkgo with meals, not on an empty stomach. As I explained in chapter 9, taking it with food means your stomach lining will not be exposed to high concentrations of the extract and so will not be as irritated by it. It's the irritation of your stomach lining that makes you feel nauseous and that can cause your bowels to churn around uncomfortably.
2. Take your ginkgo with a large glass of juice or water. This will further decrease its concentration in your stomach.
3. Decrease your daily dose.

4. Cut down, or preferably cut out, all the other things in your diet and lifestyle that make your stomach more sensitive. This means alcohol, smoking, caffeine, pickled or fatty foods, and so on. This is a good idea for your general health anyway. You will be amazed at the difference it can make. At the very least don't take other stomach-irritating foods or nutritional supplements like vitamins at the same time as ginkgo extract.

5. If you are using a more highly concentrated extract (like a 50:1 extract), switch to a less concentrated one (like a 1:1 liquid extract).

6. If you are using a liquid extract, instead of taking it two or three times a day, try spreading it out to five times a day. Take the same total dose each day but in smaller portions. Have three small portions with your three meals and the other two small portions as a snack in between meals.

7. Try putting your daily dose of liquid extract into a 1.5-liter bottle of spring water in the morning and sipping from it throughout the day.

8. Try the glycerine-based liquid extract (see appendix 2 for suppliers) instead of the alcohol-based extract. It could be the alcohol in the extract that is the problem, not the medicinal substances.

9. Try a flavored extract instead of a plain one (see appendix 2). It may be more palatable for you.

10. Although it's a strong spice, ginger is a powerful remedy for nausea. Some doctors recommend it for patients who have nausea due to chemotherapy, which is one of the

worst kinds of nausea. You can get ginger at your grocery store in the spice section or raw in the produce department. Make a cup of tea with two teaspoons of the grated or powdered root. A glass of ginger ale will also provide the right dose. In some people, though, ginger can cause heartburn.

Side Effect 2: Headaches

In a 1991 study of 303 patients taking ginkgo, headache was the side effect that was most prominent. 1.3 percent of the patients reported headache, compared with 0.3 percent of those taking a placebo.[3] What's interesting about this particular side effect is that in many patients ginkgo is actually effective in *treating* headache. So that it should cause headache in some patients is curious indeed.

I can offer two explanations. First, it's surprising but true that any medication that relieves a headache, if taken regularly for a prolonged period, can turn around and cause a headache. This is due to a sort of "rebound" effect, in which the body reacts against the medication, becoming more easily triggered to start up another headache. Neurologists see many patients with this problem, who have one migraine after another and are unaware that the drugs they are taking to relieve their headaches are actually setting off their next ones. Perhaps this is why ginkgo can both treat headaches and cause them.

The second explanation is related to the fact that ginkgo

contains many active ingredients. Some of them cause dilation of small blood vessels throughout the body. People prone to migraines are very sensitive to anything that causes even a tiny bit of dilation of their blood vessels. Other ingredients in ginkgo, though, can relieve migraines, through a variety of means.

So whether ginkgo causes or relieves a headache may depend on which ingredient is present in a slightly higher concentration than another in a particular extract.

If you have a history of migraines, you should probably start with a lower dose of ginkgo. If you develop headaches while taking ginkgo, I recommend that you see your doctor.

Side Effect 3: Allergic Reactions

Virtually anything can cause an allergic response, and ginkgo is no exception. Ginkgo leaf extracts contain at least seven different substances known to cause allergy in some individuals.[4] (It also contains at least eight different substances that treat allergies! See chapter 5 for more details.) The main culprits are thought to be *ginkgolic acids*. These acids, which are similar to substances found in poison ivy, are found in the highest concentrations in the pulpy fruit layer surrounding the ginkgo seed. As a result, people who pick the fruit or unwashed seeds often end up with a rash on their hands. If they're unfortunate enough to eat the fruit, they can develop inflammation in their mouths and digestive tracts.[5]

Ginkgolic acids are also found in ginkgo leaves, but in much lower concentrations. For this reason most authorities on botanical medicine do not recommend the use of crude ginkgo leaf extracts. If you use high doses of crude leaf extract, you may ingest enough ginkgolic acids to cause inflammation. The German federal health commission has therefore recommended that ginkgo leaf extracts be purified to contain a maximum of five parts per million of ginkgolic acids.[6] Standardized extracts should meet this specification.

Despite purification of extracts, allergic reactions can still occur. The commonest manifestation of an allergy to ginkgo extract is a rash. If your stomach and intestines become inflamed from allergic contact with the drug, you may also experience nausea, abdominal pain, and diarrhea. These are the same symptoms that were mentioned under "Stomach and Intestinal Symptoms," where they were ascribed to nonallergic causes. It's not always easy to tell if a side effect is due to allergy or some other cause. This is one of the reasons you should talk to your doctor as soon as possible about any side effect you experience. If a true allergic reaction develops when you're using the extract, you should stop using it. The most serious allergic reactions are those where the person's airways swell up and threaten to close off. Theoretically this reaction can occur with any drug, though there are no reports of it ever happening with ginkgo. If your lips, tongue, or throat do swell up, however, or if you have difficulty breathing, you need to call an ambulance immediately and be treated in an emergency room.

Side Effect 4: Restlessness or Irritability

In all of the studies on ginkgo, restlessness or irritability either were very uncommon as side effects or did not occur at all. Nonetheless I'm discussing them here because I've personally encountered them in two cases. These people described themselves as feeling jittery or "activated" when they used the standardized extract.

As we know from tests of mental functioning, ginkgo is not a stimulant. It does have some antidepressant effects, which may account for the fact that it seems to "activate" some people. You don't have to be depressed for an antidepressant to make you feel restless or irritable. These drugs cause specific biochemical changes in the brain of anyone who takes them. But some people are more sensitive than others to the effects of medications.

If you feel restless or irritable when you take the standardized ginkgo extract, it's probably too strong for your system to handle. You're more likely to experience other side effects, too. Decreasing the dose might help, but it's not very convenient to cut capsules in half. Decreasing the frequency with which you take it might help, but it's necessary to take it at least twice a day to keep a continuous supply of active ingredients on board. If you take only one capsule daily, you might not obtain as many of ginkgo's long-term benefits. The best solution is probably to use the less concentrated forms of ginkgo, like ginkgo leaf tea, or capsules containing the plain freeze-dried leaf powder, or the unstandardized liquid extracts in low doses. (See appendix 2 for suppliers.)

Does Ginkgo Cause Bleeding?

In the past two years, two cases have been reported in the journal *Neurology* in which patients taking ginkgo extract were discovered to have hemorrhaged into the area surrounding their brain, the subdural space.[7] In a separate report in the *New England Journal of Medicine,* a patient taking ginkgo extract experienced a small hemorrhage in his eye.[8] Did the ginkgo have anything to do with these cases of bleeding? If ginkgo was the culprit, these side effects would be the most serious ever reported for it.

The first patient was a 33-year-old woman who had been taking 120 mg of ginkgo extract daily. After about a year and a half, she began to develop increasingly severe headaches.[9] Her doctor ordered an MRI scan, which showed an abnormal collection of blood in the subdural space around her brain. She was taken to the operating room and had the blood drained off without any complications.

Nobody suspected the ginkgo, however, so she continued to take it for another six months. During this time her headaches persisted. She was referred to a neurologist, who ordered another MRI. No new bleeding was found. Wondering about the cause of the woman's previous hemorrhage, the neurologist ordered a test called a bleeding time, which measures the ability of the blood's platelets to put an end to bleeding. The results were slightly abnormal. The neurologist suspected that the ginkgo might be the cause of her abnormal platelet function and might have caused her hemorrhage many months before. He recommended that she stop taking ginkgo. A month after discontinuing ginkgo, her bleeding time was improved, but it was still not completely normal. She decided to not take ginkgo again anyway. On follow-up fifteen months later, she was well and free from headaches.

After the case report was published, a group of doctors wrote in to the journal, arguing that the ginkgo was unlikely to have caused her subdural hemorrhage.[10] Such hemorrhages are often found in people with no obvious risk factors, they reasoned, and although her bleeding time improved slightly after the ginkgo was stopped, the bleeding time test is well known to be unreliable. As a result, they said, there was no proof of any ill effect of ginkgo.

In my opinion, however, there is enough evidence to suggest that the ginkgo was at least partly the cause of this young woman's hemorrhage. Ginkgo, as I discussed in chapter 4, is known to cause a decrease in the ability of platelets to stop bleeding and blood to clot. Even though the bleeding time test is notoriously inaccurate, her results still give some support to the idea that ginkgo was affecting her clotting.

The fact that her bleeding time test result was still slightly abnormal one month after stopping the ginkgo, however, suggests that something else was affecting it, too. She may have had some subtle disease of her platelets, or perhaps she was eating a lot of wood ear mushrooms or other foods that affected them. In other words, I don't think ginkgo was the only culprit here.

The second report of a patient with a hemorrhage came about a year later.[11] In this case, a 72-year-old woman had been taking 150 mg of ginkgo extract daily for six to seven months. She then came to her doctor, complaining of dizziness and memory loss for the previous six months. A CT scan of her brain was ordered. It showed a small subdural hemorrhage, which appeared to be several months old.

In commenting on this case, the authors admitted that it was again difficult to see whether the hemorrhage had anything to do with the ginkgo. In this case, I agree with them. For one thing, it was not clear that the hemorrhage hadn't been there before the woman took the ginkgo. The hemorrhage may well have caused her initial dizziness and memory loss, symptoms the woman had then tried to treat with ginkgo.

The third case report was published at about the same time. It concerned a 70-year-old man who had been taking aspirin regularly for three years.[12] He then started to take 80 mg of ginkgo extract daily. One week later he developed a small hemorrhage in the iris of his eye. The bleeding stopped on its own, without any complications. He followed his doctor's advice to stop taking ginkgo and had no further problems.

Undoubtedly, some of the blame for the bleeding in this man's case must lie with the aspirin. But I also think it's too much of a coincidence that the bleeding occurred so soon after he started the ginkgo extract. The extract must have been partly responsible.

What does all this add up to? Ginkgo extract may well be a risk factor for hemorrhage, especially when it's combined with other drugs known to cause bleeding, like aspirin. Hence I advise against using it if you're taking such drugs, or if you have an illness affecting blood clotting (see chapter 7). I also advise anyone taking ginkgo to see their doctor if they develop severe headaches, dizziness, or other new symptoms, because of the remote risk that they may have had a hemorrhage.

We need to see this risk in perspective, however. These three cases of bleeding are the only ones ever reported, out of literally millions of patients who have taken ginkgo extract. As a comparison, ticlopidine has a rate of bleeding within the brain of 0.5 percent, and aspirin has a rate of 0.6 percent.[13] Overall, ginkgo's safety record is far better than almost any synthetic drug of any type.

Rare Side Effects

Other side effects that have been reported in less than half of one percent of patients include burning eyes and breathlessness.[14] I have personally encountered a variant of the first, in a patient who complained of red eyes but had no discomfort. It looked as though the small blood vessels in his eyes were dilated. This would make sense, since ginkgo does cause dilation of blood vessels throughout the body. When he stopped ginkgo, the problem resolved. If you experience either of these symptoms, I'd recommend that you cease taking the extract and see your doctor.

A Final Note on Side Effects

I want to emphasize again that this book is not meant to replace the care of your doctor. You should use ginkgo only under their supervision. Please remain alert for side effects and report them to your doctor immediately. You are unique, and your therapy needs individual attention and care.

Chapter 11

GROWING AND HARVESTING GINKGO

Okay. You've tried the stuff, and you like it. You don't have a serious illness that requires you to use a standardized extract. You're a down-to-earth kind of person, you're patient, and you've got a big front yard. You're the ideal person to grow your own ginkgo.

Growing ginkgo is a long-term investment. It takes about five years for it to start paying off. That's when you can start harvesting the leaves in reasonable amounts. When you grow the tree for its seeds, as many Asians do, it's an especially long-term investment. It's not for nothing that one of the Asian names for the tree is *Grandfather and grandson tree*. Ginkgo trees take about twenty years to mature and produce seeds—so a person would gather seeds from a tree their grandfather planted.[1]

Take heart, though; growing ginkgo is easy, especially if you plant saplings from a nursery. All it requires is the cost of the seeds or sapling and one afternoon of your time. Thereafter, apart from a little watering during dry spells, ginkgo is maintenance-free.

If you don't want to grow your own ginkgo but have access to ginkgos in unpolluted areas, this chapter still contains useful information for you. You'll learn how to harvest and prepare the leaves yourself and even make your own extract.

Where to Plant It

Ginkgo can grow just about anywhere in a temperate climate; all over the United States, from Florida to Washington State. They prefer it cooler, so they flourish in Canada. They have a fair amount of drought tolerance. They're not picky about soil, either, but well-drained, rich soil is always better.

If you're planting a seedling and don't know which sex it is, be certain you don't plant it next to a sidewalk or street. Some cities have ordinances against planting female ginkgo trees. The slippery and bad-smelling fruits can be a hazard for pedestrians. If you call around to nurseries, you should be able to find saplings propagated from cuttings from male trees, so you can be certain of the sex. If you're able to plant female trees in your city, however, I'd recommend you do so, since the nuts are a delicacy.

Make sure you've got room for the tree. They grow tall, up to 120 feet, and about 40 feet wide.

Growing from Seeds

If there are no female trees in your area, you can get sproutable ginkgo seeds from a seed supply house or a Chinese grocery store. Put a couple handfuls of wet peat moss or sand in a plastic sandwich bag, and bury a few ginkgo seeds in it. Leave the bag in the house at room temperature. The seeds should sprout within a few weeks if they're viable. As soon as they do, remove them from the bag and plant them in small pots, keeping the soil moist. Sun-harden the seedlings by not leaving them in the shade. After a few months in the pots, plant them out in the desired location, preferably in full sun. Avoid doing this during times of excessive cold or heat—frost can destroy ginkgo's roots if the ground is wet.

Then relax—your ginkgo tree will never need spraying or pruning. The need for raking will be minimal, too, since ginkgos drop their leaves all at one time, sometimes in a single day. If the soil's poor, fertilizing it during the growing season would be a good idea. Twice a month from spring to mid-summer would be plenty.

Harvesting and Preparing the Leaves

There are two different times to harvest ginkgo leaves, depending on which ingredients of the leaf you are trying to get the most of. If you are using ginkgo for its brain-boosting or anti-allergy effects, you need more ginkgolides, so you should harvest in September, just before the trees start to withdraw nourishment from their leaves. By October the leaves have turned yellow, and their content of ginkgolides is lower.[2] In the Southern Hemisphere, the equivalent time for harvest is in March.

If you are using ginkgo as a longevity tonic, you should wait until the leaves turn yellow before you harvest them. Their concentrations of bioflavonoids will be higher, giving stronger antioxidant or anti-aging effects.[3] The Chinese and Japanese have traditionally harvested the leaves at this time.

Harvesting the leaves from September onward does not harm the trees, since they would soon drop them anyway. Still, avoid taking more than a few leaves from young trees.

Once you've harvested and washed the leaves, you have a few different options for preparing them. The simplest is to dry them. Place them on a wire screen to allow air to circulate around them, and set them in the shade for a few days. Don't dry them in the sun, since it will cause a breakdown of the active ingredients. If your climate is too humid to dry the leaves within a few days, you can obtain a dehydrator (used for fruits and vegetables) from any large department store. Place the dried leaves in a paper bag inside an airtight, preferably lightproof container, and store them in a cool place. This will minimize air- and light-induced degradation of the active ingredients.

You can make tea with the leaves as described in chapter 9, or grind up them up and fill capsules with the powder. You can obtain empty capsules for this purpose from a health food store. Take one filled capsule three times a day.

How to Make Your Own Extract

Another way to prepare your leaves is to make a liquid extract from them. Use fresh, undried leaves. Remove the stems, and crush or grind the leaves finely. Pack a jar with them, and top it up with vodka. (In traditional Chinese medicine ginkgo leaf extracts are made with rice wine rather than vodka.) Cover and leave it for a couple of weeks, then strain it. Then it's ready for use.

The ideal way to store your liquid extract is in a dark glass container with a tightly fitting lid. Keep it in a cool place, like the refrigerator. To use the extract, measure out fifteen drops with a medicine dropper, and mix into a glass of warm water. Take three of these glasses daily. If the effect is inadequate after six weeks of treatment, increase the dose to 30 drops three times a day.

You'll find that growing and/or preparing your own ginkgo is easier than you think. It's a satisfying hobby, too. Enjoy!

Chapter 12

THE SACRED EARTH: THE ENVIRONMENTAL MESSAGE OF GINKGO

The Mind of Gaia

In a time before human time, long before the emergence of the kind of awareness we humans call consciousness, another kind of awareness began unraveling and breathing and moving about on our planet. It was a wordless awareness; or rather, it was too profound for words. Instead of the brains of individual creatures generating this awareness, its mind encompassed whole species and whole ecosystems.

Its thoughts were shaped in the forms of serpentine DNA molecules, elegant proteins, and exotic alkaloids. The synapses between the cells of this mind were the interactions between species—one giving shelter to another, one eating another, one decomposing to give life to another. Different species shared certain thoughts—certain biochemical shapes in their proteins or DNA. So a single chemical could affect many diverse species in different ways. It was as though one species would think part of one thought, and another would complete it. This is the way the mind of Gaia—the living earth—developed.

Across 200 million years, one of those thoughts has been a yearning for protection from the ravages of time. Among the many species involved in this thought, ginkgo has been the most central. As a species and as individual trees, its remarkable chemistry has enabled it to withstand the vicissitudes of time for longer than any other living thing. Ginkgo has also been a central part of Gaia's memory—it is itself a living memory of the earth the way it was 200 million years ago.

If the biosphere of our earth really works like a mind, then we too can become part of its thoughts about timelessness and memory. When we take ginkgo, it reaches down into our very cell membranes and molecules to share its thoughts. We age more slowly, and our memory improves. So in a very real way, when we take ginkgo, we participate in the mind of Gaia.

A Sacred Task

As a species, human beings have received an awesome gift. We were privileged to develop an intelligence that set us on the path to toolmaking, speech, civilization, and religion. We didn't develop all this alone. We did it while we were totally enmeshed in and supported by the vast web of life on this planet. The animals, plants, and microorganisms who fed us, provided our oxygen, and sustained the cycle of life, death, and new life for us, were all our midwives. And though we may see ourselves as separate from or in control of the web of life now, in reality we are as dependent on it as ever. So although we are privileged to be the carriers of the gift of intelligence, it is not really ours alone. It is an expression of the totality of life on this planet. It is another of the thoughts of Gaia.

Just as our intelligence has been entrusted to us by the rest of life on earth, so too the task of safekeeping the earth has been given us. We're only just beginning to understand this. Sadly, of late, we've been doing a poor job of safekeeping.

Some shining examples of what we can achieve, however, do exist. The story of ginkgo is one of them. Its survival thanks to human efforts shows the positive impact that an attitude of respectful stewardship can have on preserving the world's environment. It also shows the beneficial effects that such preservation can have on our personal health. Ginkgo helps heal our minds and bodies, and can even assist us in meditation. Similarly, the sacred task of safeguarding Gaia can help us achieve our potential on all levels—mentally, physically, and spiritually.

When we talk about self-interest as a reason for conservation, then, we need to understand that our self-interest is really, in a larger sense, the self-interest of the planet, too. When we save a species from extinction, it's not we alone who benefit but the whole biosphere. It may seem to us that we are saving it because of its medicinal value to us, but in reality our action helps heal the earth itself.

Never before has all of this been so important for us to

understand as it is now. Of the eighty thousand species of plants that exist in the Amazon, dozens disappear each day. The rain forests of South America, Southeast Asia, and Africa continue to be clear-cut and burned to make way for grazing land for cattle. Priceless botanical medicines that we will never know about are slipping through our fingers.

Of course, the loss of potential medicines isn't the only reason to preserve the rain forests. We should protect them simply because they're there. This is the task that Gaia has apportioned us.

One of the most effective things you can do personally is reduce the amount of red meat that you eat. If the demand for beef went down, so would the rate of deforestation. You can also become a member of a group that lobbies for environmental concerns, like the Sierra Club or the Wilderness Society. When you take these simple steps, you become part of Gaia's immune system.

The healing forces of the earth can heal us. And we can return the favor.

Appendix 1

WHY THIS BOOK IS CRUELTY-FREE

As I mentioned in chapter 3, I have not cited the results of animal experiments in this book. I considered the issue carefully and came to this decision for a number of reasons.

For one thing, when I learned what some of these experiments consisted of, I was dismayed. In one study, for example, rats were isolated and kept in refrigerators for five days, in order to stress them. They were then given ginkgo, then were killed, and their brains were examined to determine the amounts of various receptors in them. No comfort was given these rats, since the whole idea was to stress them as much as possible.

In another study, guinea pigs had one of their ears cut out. This produced a state of dizziness. They were then immobilized in harnesses that tilted their heads in different directions, making them feel as though they were spinning. They were then given ginkgo to see if this would stop their eyes from jerking back and forth in response to their dizziness.

Again, no pain relief or antinausea medications were given, since that would have invalidated the results.

In another experiment, hungry rats were presented with food but were given electric shocks when they tried to eat it. Then they were given ginkgo to see if it would help them learn to avoid the food more quickly.

These kind of studies are awful to read about. Most people would be horrified if they knew about the amount of suffering inflicted on animals for the sake of the medicines they take, or the lipsticks or shampoos they use. Each year, between 25 and 50 million animals are killed in laboratory experiments in the United States alone.[1] They are subjected to many painful procedures, including being burned, poisoned, cut open, and dismembered while fully conscious. As in the studies on ginkgo, they are often provided with no anaesthesia, since that would interfere with the functioning of their bodies and render the results of the experiments invalid.

The most scandalous part of this situation is that almost all of the information that animal studies provide us can be obtained in cruelty-free ways. We now have the technology—the use of tissue cultures, computer modeling, sophisticated biochemical analyses, noninvasive studies of humans, and other methods—that in most cases we no longer need animal experiments.

In addition, as I went through all the animal studies on ginkgo, I realized that almost none of them had actually contributed anything significant to our knowledge. The study on dizzy guinea pigs, for example, was completely useless. We already had clinical studies on humans that proved that ginkgo helps relieve dizziness. Learning that it helps relieve dizziness in guinea pigs who have had their ears cut out helps no one. All that study achieved was that a scientist got his name published.

The few experiments that have contributed a smidgeon to our knowledge could have been replaced by studies of humans. The study of cold-stressed rats, for example, could have been replaced by a study using a technique called positron-emission tomography (PET) scanning, in which the receptor numbers in human brains can be measured noninvasively. The human subjects would not have had to be isolated or refrigerated; instead the researchers could have paid people who are under stress—like university students studying for finals—to be their subjects. The results would then have been much more valuable than the experiment on rats, because rat brains are very different from human brains anyway.

In fact, very few animal studies of any type have provided information that can be reliably applied to humans. The physiology of animals is so different from humans' that experimenting on them just doesn't make much sense. They don't get the same diseases that we do, and they respond quite differently to our drugs.[2] In the case of ginkgo, for example, although tests show ginkgo has no adverse effect on liver enzymes in humans, it has quite strong effects on liver enzymes in mice.[3] Animals also have different types of receptors for platelet-activating factor, so ginkgolides affect them very differently from humans.[4]

Relying on the results of animal studies can actually be dangerous, putting humans at serious risk for injury. Pregnant animals, for instance, have traditionally been used to determine if new drugs cause birth defects. But many drugs that were tested on animals and declared safe then went on to tragically cause serious birth defects in humans. The animal tests had been worse than useless, since they gave a false sense of security. One of the leading current reference books on drug safety in pregnancy totally omits the results of animal tests, relying only on human data.[5]

Animal experiments go on, though, because they're often quicker, easier, and cheaper, and researchers are accustomed to them. In rare cases animal experiments are justifiable, since they provide valuable information for healing humans that can be obtained in no other way. But most animal experiments are pointless and, I believe, morally bankrupt. Many other physicians and scientists agree with me. I have therefore chosen not to honor animal researchers by citing their names in this book.

Several organizations are now devoted to approaching this issue in a moderate way, allowing for the occasional justifiable use of animals in experiments while sponsoring research on developing and implementing alternatives to animal testing. Their membership includes many notable scientists and laypeople.

For more information on animal experimentation and how you can help end it, visit the website of the American Antivivisection Society at www.aavs.org. Or you can contact them at:

The American Antivivisection Society
801 Old York Road, #204
Jenkintown, PA 19046-1685
Phone: 1-215-887-0816

Membership is $20 per year ($10 for students) and includes a magazine subscription.

Other websites worth visiting are the Humane Society of the United States at www.hsus.org, the Johns Hopkins Center for Alternatives to Animal Testing at www.sph.jhu.edu/~altweb/, and the Fund for the Replacement of Animals in Medical Experiments at: www.frame-uk.demon.co.uk/

Appendix 2

SUPPLIERS OF GINKGO

Extracts and Leaves

Most health food stores, grocery chains, drugstores, and even discount stores in the United States now carry ginkgo extracts. Here's a list of some other retail sources, the types of products they carry, their Internet addresses, and their phone, fax, and street addresses if they supplied them. A listing here does not necessarily mean that I endorse their particular products or services.

Nonstandardized liquid extracts, glycerine-based extracts, and flavored extracts, as well as ground-up, freeze-dried leaves in capsules, which are also nonstandardized, are available from:

Eclectic Institute
P.O. Box 936
Sandy, OR 97055-9549
Phone: 1-800-332-4372
Fax: 1-503-668-3227
www.eclecticherb.com

High-potency standardized capsules, 140 mg:

New Gaia Products
2934 Upshur Street
San Diego, CA 92106
Fax: 1-619-222-9701

Discounted standardized capsules:

Nutrition Headquarters, Inc.
One Nutrition Plaza
Carbondale, IL 62901-8825
Fax: 1-618-529-4553

Extra–high potency standardized capsules, 180 mg:

Raytech
P.O. Box 27740
Las Vegas, NV 89102
Phone: 1-800-838-5898 or 1-805-822-7567
Fax: 1-805-822-0869
http://raytech.simplenet.com

Discounted standardized capsules:

Smart Basics
Phone: 1-800-878-6520 or 1-415-749-3990
Fax: 1-415-351-1348
www.smartbasic.com

Ginkgold, the original standardized Schwabe capsules from Europe:

Springtime, Inc.
www.springtimeinc.com

Ginkgoton Tea, or ginkgo extract in tea form. Each tea-bag contains the equivalent of one capsule of standardized extract.

Trademark Distributing, Inc.
15500 Erwin Street, Suite 1001A
Van Nuys, CA 91411
Phone: 1-800-870-7590
Fax: 1-818-901-2837
http://home.earthlink.net/~trademarkinc/

Extracts and dry leaves, imported from China:

U.C. Medicine, Inc.
350 Fifth Avenue, Suite 4517
New York, NY 10118
Phone: 1-212-736-6211
Fax: 1-212-736-6213
www.uschinatrade.com

Ginkgo Trees Delivered

Full-size saplings and bonsai ginkgos; will ship internationally. Priced from four to twenty U.S. dollars per tree.

Evergreen Gardenworks
P.O. Box 1357
Ukiah, CA 95482
Phone: 1-707-462-8909

Appendix 3

HOW TO FIND A DOCTOR WHO PRACTICES HOLISTIC MEDICINE

Holistic Medicine

See chapter 7 for a discussion of what holistic medicine is all about. To locate a medical doctor in your area who practices according to the principles of holistic medicine, call or write:

American Holistic Medical Association
6728 Old McLean Village Drive
McLean, VA 22101-3906
Phone: 1-703-556-9728 (patient information)
www.ahmaholistic.com

For five dollars, you will be sent a listing of holistic physicians across the United States. Please allow four to six weeks.

Naturopathic Medicine

Naturopaths, or N.D.'s, have kept alive a lot of natural healing techniques that otherwise might have been left by the wayside and now offer them as an alternative to conventional medicine. They employ a variety of treatments, including nutritional therapy, herbalism, homeopathy, acupuncture, and physical manipulation. They are not allowed to prescribe conventional drugs, but most of them would prefer not to anyway. Naturopaths are now regulated in many states of the United States. In the past the standards for naturopathic education were poor, but recently they have improved to a point where they are coming closer to those of conventional medicine.

Naturopathic medicine is particularly good for treating chronic illnesses, where conventional medicine has failed. But naturopaths are usually less adept at diagnosis than conventional doctors. To get a firm diagnosis, you're better off seeing a conventional doctor or a holistic doctor (see above) before consulting a naturopath. Unfortunately, only a few insurance companies will pay for their services.

To locate a good naturopathic physician in your area, contact:

American Association of Naturopathic Physicians
2366 Eastlake Avenue East, Suite 322
Seattle, WA 98102
Phone: 1-206-827-6035
Fax: 1-206-323-7612

For five dollars, they'll mail you some brochures on naturopathic medicine, along with a list of licensed naturopaths across the United States.

Longevity Specialists

For more information on life extension therapies, or to locate a physician near you who specializes in this field, visit the website of the American College for the Advancement of Medicine at www.acam.org. Or you can write to:

The American College for the Advancement of Medicine
23121 Verdugo Drive, Suite 204
Laguna Hills, CA 92653

Smart Drugs

For more information on nootropics, or smart drugs, or to locate a physician near you with a special interest in them, visit the website of the Cognitive Enhancement Research Institute at: www.ceri.com

Appendix 4

FOR THE HEALTH PROFESSIONAL: IMPORTANT ARTICLES ON GINKGO

Here are some of the more easily accessible English-language references on ginkgo:

J. Kleijnen and P. Knipschild. Ginkgo biloba. *Lancet* 340 (1992): 1136–39.

P. L. Le Bars et al. A placebo-controlled, double-blind, randomized trial of an extract of Ginkgo biloba for dementia. *Journal of the American Medical Association* 267, no. 16 (1997): 1327–32.

German Federal Commission E Monograph: Ginkgo (1994). Available online from the American Botanical Council at: www.herbalgram.org

REFERENCES

Chapter 1. How Ginkgo Can Help You

1. See chapter 3 for details.
2. Ibid.
3. F. Jung et al., [Effect of Ginkgo biloba on fluidity of blood and peripheral microcirculation in volunteers,] *Arzneimittel-Forschung* 40, no. 5 (1990): 589–93; S. Witte, I. Anadere, and E. Walitza, [Improvement of hemorheology with Ginkgo biloba extract. Decreasing a cardiac risk factor,] *Fortschritte der Medizin* 110, no. 13 (1992): 247–50; M. Auguet et al., [Pharmacological bases of the vascular impact of Ginkgo biloba extract,] *Presse Medicale* 15, no. 31 (1986): 1524–28; and P. Koltringer et al., [Microcirculation and viscoelasticity of the blood with Ginkgo biloba extract. A placebo-controlled, randomized double-blind study,] *Perfusion* 1 (1989): 28–30.
4. Quoted in G. Halpern, *Ginkgo: A Practical Guide* (New York: Avery, 1998), p. 85.

5. Z. Subhan and I. Hindmarch, The psychopharmacological effects of Ginkgo biloba extract in normal healthy volunteers, *International Journal of Clinical Pharmacology Research* 4, no. 2 (1984): 89–93; and I. Hindmarch, [Activity of Ginkgo biloba extract on short-term memory,] *Presse Medicale* 15, no. 31 (1986): 1592–94.

6. F. Kunkel, EEG profile of three different extractions of Ginkgo biloba, *Neuropsychobiology* 27 (1993): 40–45.

7. H. V. Semlitsch et al., Cognitive psychophysiology in nootropic drug research: Effects of Ginkgo biloba on event-related potentials (P300) in age-associated memory impairment, *Pharmacopsychiatry* 28, no. 4 (1995): 134–42; G. S. Rai, C. Shovlin, and K. A. Wesnes, A double-blind, placebo-controlled study of Ginkgo biloba extract ("Tanakan") in elderly outpatients with mild to moderate memory impairment, *Current Medical Research and Opinion* 12, no. 6 (1991): 350–55; and H. Allain et al., Effect of two doses of Ginkgo biloba extract (Egb 761) on the dual-coding test in elderly subjects, *Clinical Therapeutics* 15, no. 3 (1993): 549–58.

8. B. Gessner, A. Voelp, and M. Klasser, [Study of the long-term action of a Ginkgo biloba extract on vigilance and mental performance as determined by means of quantitative pharmaco-EEG and psychometric measurements,] *Arzneimittel-Forschung* 35, no. 9 (1985): 1459–65; also see note 6 above.

9. See chapter 4 for details.

10. Ibid.

11. See chapter 5 for details.

12. Ibid.

13. Ibid.

14. J. Kleijnen and P. Knipschild, Ginkgo for cerebral insufficiency, *British Journal of Clinical Pharmacology* 34 (1992): 352–58; J. Kleijnen and P. Knipschild, Ginkgo biloba, *Lancet* 340 (1992): 1136–39; B. Schneider, [Ginkgo biloba extract in peripheral arterial diseases. Meta-analysis of controlled clinical studies,] *Arzneimittel-Forschung* 42, no. 4 (1992): 428–36; and E. Ernst, [Ginkgo biloba in treatment of intermittent claudication. A systematic research based on controlled studies in the literature,] *Fortschritte der Medizin* 114, no. 8 (1996): 85–87.

15. J. Kleijnen and P. Knipschild, Ginkgo biloba, *Lancet* 340 (1992): 1136–39.

16. See note 5 above.

17. Ibid.

18. F. Eckmann, [Cerebral insufficiency—treatment with Ginkgo biloba extract. Time of onset of effect in a double-blind study with 60 inpatients,] *Fortschritte der Medizin* 108, no. 29 (1990): 557–60.

19. P. L. Le Bars et al., A placebo-controlled, double-blind, randomized trial of an extract of Ginkgo biloba for dementia, *Journal of the American Medical Association* 278, no. 16 (1997): 1327–32.

20. J. Kleijnen and P. Knipschild, Ginkgo for cerebral insufficiency, *British Journal of Clinical Pharmacology* 34 (1992): 352–58.

21. A. Pietschmann, B. Kuklinski, and A. Otterstein, [Protection from UV-light-induced oxidative stress by nutritional radical scavengers,] *Zeitschrift für die Gesamte Innere Medizin und Ihre Grenzgebiete* 47, no. 11 (1992): 518–22; and E. Dumont et al., UV-C irradiation-induced peroxidative degradation of microsomal fatty acids and proteins: Protection by an extract of Ginkgo biloba L, *Free Radical Biology and Medicine* 13, no. 3 (1992): 197–203.

22. G. Halpern, *Ginkgo: A Practical Guide* (New York: Avery, 1998), p. 44.

Chapter 2. What Is Ginkgo?

1. P. Del Tredici, Ginkgos and multituberculates: Evolutionary interactions in the tertiary, *Biosystems* 22, no. 4 (1989): 327–39.

2. W. Schmid, Ginkgo thrives, *Nature* 386 (1997): 755.

3. Quoted in J. Kleijnen and P. Knipschild, Ginkgo for cerebral insufficiency, *British Journal of Clinical Pharmacology* 34 (1992): 352–58; and E. Masood, "Medicinal plants threatened by over-use," *Nature* 385 (1997): 570.

4. P. Brevoort, The US botanical market: An overview, *HerbalGram* 36 (1996).

5. See note 2 above.

Chapter 3. Ginkgo—The Brain Booster

1. Z. Subhan and I. Hindmarch, The psychopharmacological effects of Ginkgo biloba extract in normal healthy volunteers, *International Journal of Clinical Pharmacology Research* 4, no. 2 (1984): 89–93.

2. I. Hindmarch, [Activity of Ginkgo biloba extract on short-term memory,] *Presse Medicale* 15, no. 31 (1986): 1592–94.

3. G. S. Rai, C. Shovlin, and K. A. Wesnes, A double-blind, placebo-controlled study of Ginkgo biloba extract ("Tanakan") in elderly outpatients with mild to moderate memory impairment, *Current Medical Research and Opinion* 12, no. 6 (1991): 350–55; B. Gessner, A. Voelp, and M. Klasser, [Study of the long-term action of a Ginkgo biloba extract on vigilance and mental performance as determined by means of quantitative pharmaco-EEG and psychometric measurements,] *Arzneimittel-Forschung* 35, no. 9 (1985): 1459–65; H. Allain et al., Effects of two doses of Ginkgo biloba extract (EGb 761) on the dual-coding test in elderly subjects, *Clinical Therapeutics* 15, no. 3 (1993): 549–58; and H. V. Semlitsch et al., Cognitive psychophysiology in nootropic drug research: Effects of Ginkgo biloba on event-related potentials (P300) in age-associated memory impairment, *Pharmacopsychiatry* 28, no. 4 (1995): 134–42.

4. See G. S. Rai in note 3 above.

5. See H. V. Semlitsch in note 3 above.

6. F. W. Funfgeld, Ginkgo biloba extracts [letter], *Lancet* (1990): 476.

7. J. Pincemail and C. Deby, [Antiradical properties of Ginkgo biloba extract,] *Presse Medicale* 15, no. 31 (1986): 1475–79; S. A. Barth et al., Influences of Ginkgo biloba on cyclosporin A induced lipid peroxidation in human liver microsomes in comparison to vitamin E, glutathione, and N-acetylcysteine, *Biochemical Pharmacology* 41, no. 10 (1991): 1521–26; M. Diwok, B. Kublinski, and B. Ernst, [Superoxide dismutase activity of Ginkgo biloba extract,] *Zeitschrift für die Gesamte Innere Medizin und Ihre Grenzgebiete* 47, no. 7 (1992): 308–11; W. Gsell et al., Interaction of neuroprotective substances with human brain superoxide dismutase. An in vitro study, *Journal of Neural Transmission* Suppl. 45 (1995): 271–79; K. Kose and P. Dogan, Lipoperoxidation induced by hydrogen peroxide in human erythrocyte membranes. 2. Comparison of the antioxidant effect of Ginkgo biloba extract (EGb 761) with those of water-soluble and lipid-soluble antioxidants, *Journal of International Medical Research* 23, no. 1 (1995): 9–18; and D. M. Warburton, Ginkgo biloba extract and cognitive decline [letter], *British Journal of Clinical Pharmacology* 36, no. 2 (1993): 137.

8. D. M. Warburton, [Clinical psychopharmacology of Ginkgo biloba extract,] *Presse Medicale* 15, no. 31 (1986): 1595–1604.

9. P. L. Le Bars et al., A placebo-controlled, double-blind, randomized trial of an extract of Ginkgo biloba for

dementia, *Journal of the American Medical Association* 278, no. 16 (1997): 1327–32.

10. S. Kanowski et al., Proof of efficacy of the Ginkgo biloba special extract EGb 761 in outpatients suffering from mild to moderate degenerative dementia of the Alzheimer type or multi-infarct dementia, *Pharmacopsychiatry* 29, no. 2 (1996): 47–56.

11. Ibid.; and J. Haase, P. Halama, and R. Horr, [Effectiveness of brief infusions with Ginkgo biloba special extract EGb 761 in dementia of the vascular and Alzheimer type,] *Zeitschrift für Gerontologie und Geriatrie* 29, no. 4 (1996): 302–9.

12. E. W. Funfgeld, A natural and broad spectrum nootropic substance for the treatment of SDAT—the Ginkgo biloba extract, *Progress in Clinical and Biological Research* 317 (1989): 1247–60.

13. *Physicians' Desk Reference,* 52nd ed. (New Jersey: Medical Economics Company, 1998).

14. F. Jung et al., Effect of Ginkgo biloba on fluidity of blood and peripheral microcirculation in volunteers, *Arzneimittel-Forschung* 40, no. 5 (1990): 589–93; and S. Witte, I. Anadere, and E. Walitza, [Improvement of hemorheology with Ginkgo biloba extract. Decreasing a cardiac risk factor,] *Fortschritte der Medizin* 110, no. 13 (1992): 247–50.

15. M. Auguet et al., [Pharmacological bases of the vascular impact of Ginkgo biloba extract,] *Presse Medicale* 15, no. 31 (1986): 1524–28; and P. Koltringer et al., [Microcir-

culation and viscoelasticity of the blood with Ginkgo biloba extract. A placebo-controlled, randomized double-blind study,] *Perfusion* 1 (1989): 28–30.

16. K. Schaffler and P. W. Reeh, [Double-blind study of the hypoxia protective effect of a standardized Ginkgo biloba preparation after repeated administration in healthy subjects,] *Arzneimittel-Forschung* 35, no. 8 (1985): 1283–86.

17. J. Kleijnen and P. Knipschild, Ginkgo for cerebral insufficiency, *British Journal of Clinical Pharmacology* 34 (1992): 352–58.

18. See note 7 above.

19. P. F. Smith, K. Maclennan, and C. L. Darlington, The neuroprotective properties of the Ginkgo biloba leaf: A review of the possible relationship to platelet-activating factor (PAF), *Journal of Ethnopharmacology* 50, no. 3 (1996): 131–39.

20. G. Lagrue, A. Behar, and A. Maurel, [Edematous syndromes caused by capillary hyperpermeability. Diffuse angioedema,] *Journal des Maladies Vasculaires* 14, no. 3 (1989): 231–35.

21. Quoted in G. Halpern, *Ginkgo: A Practical Guide* (New York: Avery, 1998), p. 85.

Chapter 4. Ginkgo—The Longevity Tonic

1. D. Ornish, *Dr. Dean Ornish's Program for Reversing Heart Disease* (New York: Ballantine, 1990).

2. F. Clostre, [From the body to the cell membrane: The different levels of pharmacologic action of Ginkgo biloba extract,] *Presse Medicale* 15, no. 31 (1986): 1529–38.

3. A Bruel et al., Effects of Ginkgo biloba extract on glucose transport and glycogen synthesis of cultured smooth muscle cells from pig aorta, *Pharmacological Research* 21, no. 4 (1989): 421–29.

4. K. Chen, W. Q. Zhou, and P. Gao, [Clinical study on the effect of the shuxuening tablet in treatment of coronary heart disease,] *Chung-Kuo Chung Hsi i Chieh Ho Tsa Chih* 16, no. 1 (1996): 24–26; R. Kenzelmann and F. Kade, [Limitation of the deterioration of lipid parameters by a standardized garlic-ginkgo combination product. A multicenter placebo-controlled double-blind study,] *Arzneimittel-Forschung* 43, no. 9 (1993): 978–81; and H. Hammerl et al., [Effect of an extract from Ginkgo biloba L. on metabolites of lipids and carbohydrates,] *Wiener Medizinische Wochenschrift* 121 (1971): 572–74.

5. See note 2 above.

6. M. Auguet et al., [Pharmacological bases of the vascular impact of Ginkgo biloba extract,] *Presse Medicale* 15, no. 31 (1986): 1524–28.

7. S. Witte, I. Anadere, and E. Walitza, [Improvement of hemorheology with Ginkgo biloba extract. Decreasing a cardiac risk factor,] *Fortschritte der Medizin* 110, no. 13 (1992): 247–50; and F. Jung et al., [Effect of Ginkgo biloba on fluidity of blood and peripheral microcirculation in volunteers,] *Arzneimittel-Forschung* 40, no. 5 (1990): 589–93.

8. K. Chen, W. Q. Zhou, and P. Gao, [Clinical study on the effect of the shuxuening tablet in treatment of coronary heart disease,] *Chung-Kuo Chung Hsi i Chieh Ho Tsa Chih* 16, no. 1 (1996): 24–26.

9. L. W. Way, ed., *Current Surgical Diagnosis and Treatment,* 10th ed. (New Jersey: Prentice-Hall, 1994), p. 741.

10. J. Blume, M. Kieser, and U. Holscher, [Placebo-controlled double-blind study of the effectiveness of Ginkgo biloba special extract EGb 761 in trained patients with intermittent claudication,] *Vasa* 25, no. 3 (1996): 265–74; E. Ernst, [Ginkgo biloba in treatment of intermittent claudication: A systematic research based on controlled studies in the literature,] *Fortschritte der Medizin* 114, no. 8 (1996): 85–87; B. Schneider, [Ginkgo biloba extract in peripheral arterial diseases. Meta-analysis of controlled clinical studies,] *Arzneimittel-Forschung* 42, no. 4 (1992): 428–36; G. J. Thompson et al., A clinical trial of Ginkgo biloba extract in patients with intermittent claudication, *International Angiology* 9, no. 2 (1990): 75–78; U. Bauer, [Ginkgo biloba extract in the treatment of arteriopathy of the lower extremities. A 65-week trial,] *Presse Medicale* 15, no. 31 (1986): 1546–49; and U. Bauer, [6-month double-blind randomized clinical trial of Ginkgo biloba extract versus placebo in two parallel groups in patients suffering from peripheral arterial insufficiency,] *Arzneimittel-Forschung* 34, no. 6 (1984): 716–20.

11. See J. Blume, M. Kieser, and U. Holscher in note 10 above.

12. F. Saudreau et al., [Efficacy of an extract of Ginkgo biloba in the treatment of chronic obliterating arteriopathies of the lower limb at stage III of the Fontaine classification,] *Journal des Maladies Vasculaires* 14 (1989): 177–82.

13. J. Kleijen and P. Knipschild, Ginkgo biloba, *Lancet* 340, no. 7 (1992): 1136–39; and H. Drabaek et al., [The effect of Ginkgo biloba extract in patients with intermittent claudication,] *Ugeskr Laeger* 158, no. 27 (1996): 3928–31.

14. Quoted in Physicians' Committee for Responsible Medicine Nutrition Factsheet, *Research on the Major Killers of Americans* (1998), available at www.pcrm.org

15. I. Emerit, N. Oganesian et al., Clastogenic factors in the plasma of Chernobyl accident recovery workers: Anticlastogenic effect of Ginkgo biloba extract, *Radiation Research* 144, no. 2 (1995): 198–205; and I. Emerit, R. Arutyunyan et al., Radiation-induced clastogenic factors: Anticlastogenic effect of Ginkgo biloba extract, *Free Radical Biology and Medicine* 18, no. 6 (1995): 985–91.

16. See I. Emerit, R. Arutyunyan et al. in note 15 above.

17. See I. Emerit, N. Oganesian et al. in note 15 above.

18. H. Itokawa et al., Antitumor principles from Ginkgo biloba L, *Chemical and Pharmaceutical Bulletin* 35, no. 7 (1987): 3016–20; and S. M. Beckstrom-Sternberg and J. A. Duke, Chemicals and their biological activities in: Ginkgo biloba L. (Ginkoaceae), in *Phytochemeco Database* (U.S. Department of Agriculture, 1998).

19. H. Itokawa et al., A quantitative structure-activity relationship for antitumor activity of long-chain phenols from

Ginkgo biloba L, *Chemical and Pharmaceutical Bulletin* 37, no. 6 (1989): 1619–21.

20. See S. M. Beckstrom-Sternberg and J. A. Duke in note 18 above.

21. P. E. Poubelle et al., Platelet-activating factor (PAF-acether) enhances the concomitant production of tumor necrosis factor-alpha and interleukin-1 by subsets of human monocytes, *Immunology* 72, no. 2 (1991): 181–87.

22. A. Pietschmann, B. Kuklinski, and A. Otterstein, [Protection from UV-light-induced oxidative stress by nutritional radical scavengers,] *Zeitschrift für die Gesamte Innere Medizin und Ihre Grenzgebiete* 47, no. 11 (1992): 518–22.

23. E. Dumont et al., UV-C irradiation-induced peroxidative degradation of microsomal fatty acids and proteins: Protection by an extract of Ginkgo biloba L, *Free Radical Biology and Medicine* 13, no. 3 (1992): 197–203.

24. G. Halpern, *Ginkgo: A Practical Guide* (New York: Avery, 1998).

25. D. A. Lebuisson, L. Leroy, and G. Rigal, [Treatment of senile macular degeneration with Ginkgo biloba extract. A preliminary double-blind drug vs. placebo study,] *Presse Medicale* 15, no. 31 (1986): 1556–58.

26. A. Raabe, M. Raabe, and P. Ihm, [Therapeutic follow-up using automatic perimetry in chronic cerebroretinal ischemian elderly patients. Prospective double-blind study with graduated-dose Ginkgo biloba treatment (EGb 761),] *Klinische Monatsblätter für Augenheilkunde* 199, no. 6 (1991): 432–38; and P. Lanthony and J. P. Cosson, [The

course of color vision in early diabetic retinopathy treated with Ginkgo biloba extract. A preliminary double-blind versus placebo study,] *Journal Français d'Ophthalmologie* 11, no. 10 (1988): 671–74.

27. B. Mayer, [Multicenter randomized double-blind drug versus placebo study of the treatment of tinnitus with Ginkgo biloba extract,] *Presse Medicale* 15, no. 31 (1986): 1562–64.

28. B. Mayer, [A multicenter study of tinnitus. epidemiology and therapy,] *Annales d'Oto-Laryngologie et de Chirurgie Cervico-Faciale* 103, no. 3 (1986): 185–88.

29. K. M. Holgers, A. Axelsson, and I. Pringle, Ginkgo biloba extract for the treatment of tinnitus, *Audiology* 33, no. 2 (1994): 85–92.

30. C. F. Claussen, [Diagnostic and practical value of cranio-corpography in vertiginous syndromes,] *Presse Medicale* 15, no. 31 (1986): 1565–68; and J. P. Haguenauer et al., [Treatment of equilibrium disorders with Ginkgo biloba extract. A multicenter double-blind drug versus placebo study,] *Presse Medicale* 15, no. 31 (1986): 1569–72.

31. C. Dubreuil, [Therapeutic trial in acute cochlear deafness. A comparative study of Ginkgo biloba extract and nicergoline,] *Presse Medicale* 15, no. 31 (1986): 1559–61.

32. Quoted in Halpern, *Ginkgo;* pp. 123–24.

Chapter 5. Ginkgo Heals Asthma, Allergies, Diabetes, PMS, and More

1. D. P. Reid, *Chinese Herbal Medicine* (Boston: Shambhala, 1987), pp. 11–12; and M. Porkert, *Chinese Medicine* (New York: Henry Holt, 1990), p. 238.

2. N. M. Roberts et al., Effect of a PAF antagonist, BN52063, on antigen-induced, acute, and late-onset cutaneous responses in atopic subjects, *Journal of Allergy and Clinical Immunology* 82, no. 2 (1988): 236–41; and C. P. Page, The role of platelet activating factor in allergic respiratory disease, *British Journal of Clinical Pharmacology* 30, Suppl. 1 (1990): 99S–106S.

3. P. Guinot et al., Effect of BN 52063, a specific PAF-acether antagonist, on bronchial provocation test to allergens in asthmatic patients. A preliminary study, *Prostaglandins* 34, no. 5 (1987): 723–31.

4. H. Wilkens et al., [Effect of the platelet-activating factor antagonist BN 52063 on exertional asthma,] *Pneumologie* 44, Suppl. 1 (1990): 347–48.

5. P. Guinot et al., Inhibition of PAF-acether induced weal and flare reaction in man by a specific PAF antagonist, *Prostaglandins* 32, no. 1 (1986): 160–63; K. F. Chung et al., Effect of a ginkgolide mixture (BN 52063) in antagonizing skin and platelet responses to platelet activating factor in man, *Lancet* 331, no. 8527 (1987): 248–51; also see N. M. Roberts et al., in note 2 above.

6. M. B. Taylor, Platelet-activating factor- and leukotriene B4-induced release of lactoferrin from blood neutrophils of atopic and nonatopic individuals, *Journal of Allergy and Clinical Immunology* 86, no. 5 (1990): 740–48.

7. S. M. Beckstrom-Sternberg and J. A. Duke, Chemicals and their biological activities in: Ginkgo biloba L. (Ginkoaceae), in *Phytochemeco Database* (U.S. Department of Agriculture, 1998).

8. R. Long, R. Yin, and Y. Zhen, [Partial purification and analysis of allergenicity, immunogenicity of Ginkgo biloba L. Pollen,] *Hua-Hsi i Ko Ta Hsueh Hsueh Pao* 23, no. 4 (1992): 429–32.

9. See chapter 10 for details.

10. P. Lanthony and J. P. Cosson, [The course of color vision in early diabetic retinopathy treated with Ginkgo biloba extract. A preliminary double-blind versus placebo study,] *Journal Français d'Ophthalmologie* 11, no. 10 (1988): 671–74.

11. I. W. Husstedt et al., Progression of distal symmetric polyneuropathy during diabetes mellitus: Clinical, neurophysiological, haemorheological changes and self-rating scales of patients, *European Neurology* 37, no. 2 (1997): 90–94.

12. Dr. Willmar Schwabe Arzneimittel [d.m.], *Tebonin Forte* (detail manual); Dr. Willmar Schwabe quoted in C. Hobbs. *Ginkgo: Elixir of Youth* (Capitola, CA: Botanica Press, 1991).

13. A. Tamborini and R. Taurelle, [Value of standardized Ginkgo biloba extract (EGb 761) in the management of congestive symptoms of premenstrual syndrome] *Revue Française de Gynécologie et d'Obstétrique* 88, nos. 7–9 (1993): 447–57.

14. J. P. Roncin, F. Schwartz, and P. D'Arbigny, EGb 761 in control of acute mountain sickness and vascular reactivity to cold exposure, *Aviation Space and Environmental Medicine* 67, no. 5 (1996): 445–52; G. Lagrue, A. Behar, and A. Maurel, [Edematous syndromes caused by capillary hyperpermeability. Diffuse angioedema,] *Journal des Maladies Vasculaires* 14, no. 3 (1989): 231–35; G. Lagrue et al., [Idiopathic cyclic edema. The role of capillary hyperpermeability and its correction by Ginkgo biloba extract,] *Presse Medicale* 15, no. 31 (1986): 1550–53; and D. Hannequin, A. Thibert, and Y. Vaschalde, [Development of a model to study the anti-edema properties of Ginkgo biloba extract,] *Presse Medicale* 15, no. 31 (1986): 1575–76.

15. Y. Mandi et al., Effect of the platelet-activating factor antagonist BN 52021 on human natural killer cell cytotoxicity, *International Archives of Allergy and Applied Immunology* 88, nos. 1–2 (1989): 222–24; and B. J. Liu, H. T. Zhang, and M. R. Zheng, [Effect of BN 52021 on platelet activating factor induced aggregation of psoriatic polymorphonuclear neutrophils,] *Chung-Hua i Hsueh Tsa Chih* 74, no. 6 (1994): 370–72, 392.

16. S. J. Kim et al., Effects of flavonoids of Ginkgo biloba on proliferation of human skin fibroblasts, *Skin Pharmacology* 10, no. 4 (1997): 200–5.

17. K. Osawa et al., The inhibitory effect of plant extracts on the collagenolytic activity and cytotoxicity of human gingival fibroblasts by Porphomonas gingivalis crude enzyme, *Bulletin of Tokyo Dental College* 32, no. 1 (1991): 1–7.

18. S. A. Barth et al., Influences of Ginkgo biloba on cyclosporin A induced lipid peroxidation in human liver microsomes in comparison to vitamin E, glutathione and N-acetylcysteine, *Biochemical Pharmacology* 41, no. 10 (1991): 1521–26.

19. W. Li, Q. T. Dai, and Z. E. Liu, [Preliminary study on early fibrosis of chronic hepatitis B treated with Ginkgo biloba Composita,] *Chung-Kuo Chung Hsi i Chieh Ho Tsa Chih* 15, no. 10 (1995): 593–95.

Chapter 6. Why Most Doctors Know Nothing About Herbs

1. *Physicians' Desk Reference,* 51st ed. (New Jersey: Medical Economics Company, 1997), p. 2318.

2. P. L. Le Bars et al., A placebo-controlled, double-blind, randomized trial of an extract of Ginkgo biloba for dementia, *Journal of the American Medical Association* 278, no. 16 (1997): 1327–32.

3. A. Weil, *Health and Healing* (Boston: Houghton Mifflin, 1983), pp. 99–102.

4. Anonymous, Ginkgo biloba extract: Over 5 million prescriptions a year [letter], *Lancet* (1989): 1513–14.

5. U. Stein, Ginkgo biloba extracts [letter], *Lancet* 335, no. 8687 (1990): 475–76.

Chapter 7. Using Ginkgo Safely

1. J. C. Duche et al., Effect of Ginkgo biloba extract on microsomal enzyme induction, *International Journal of Clinical Pharmacology Research* 9, no. 3 (1989): 165–68.

2. M. Rosenblatt and J. Mindel, Spontaneous hyphema associated with ingestion of Ginkgo biloba extract, *New England Journal of Medicine* 336, no. 15 (1997): 1108.

3. American Botanical Council (trans.), *German Federal Commission E Monograph: Ginkgo* (1994), available online at www.herbalgram.org

4. W. Deberdt, Interaction between psychological and pharmacological treatment in cognitive impairment, *Life Sciences* 55, nos. 25–26 (1994): 2057–66.

Chapter 8. How to Buy Ginkgo

1. K. Chen W. Q. Zhou, and P. Gao, [Clinical study on the effect of the shuxuening tablet in treatment of coronary heart disease,] *Chung-Kuo Chung Hsi i Chieh Ho Tsa Chih* 16, no 1 (1996): 24–26.

Chapter 9. How to Use Ginkgo

1. American Botanical Council (trans.), *German Federal Commission E Monograph: Ginkgo* (1994), available online at www.herbalgram.org

2. Z. Subhan and I. Hindmarch, The psychopharmacological effects of Ginkgo biloba extract in normal healthy volunteers, *International Journal of Clinical Pharmacology Research* 4, no. 2 (1984): 89–93; and I. Hindmarch, [Activity of Ginkgo biloba extract on short-term memory,] *Presse Medicale* 15, no. 31 (1986): 1592–94.

3. H. Kunkel, EEG profile of three different extractions of Ginkgo biloba, *Neuropsychobiology* 27 (1993): 40–45.

4. J. B. Fourtillan et al, [Pharmacokinetic properties of bilobalide and ginkgolides A and B in healthy subjects after intravenous and oral administration of Ginkgo biloba extract (EGb 761),] *Therapie* 50, no. 2 (1995): 137–44.

5. Ibid.

6. J. Kleijnen and P. Knipschild, Ginkgo biloba, *Lancet* 340 (1992): 1136–39.

7. See note 4 above.

8. See note 6 above.

9. See notes 2 and 3 above.

10. F. Eckmann, [Cerebral insufficiency—treatment with Ginkgo biloba extract. Time of onset of effect in a double-blind study with 60 inpatients,] *Fortschritte der Medizin* 108, no. 29 (1990): 557–60.

11. C. Hobbs, *Ginkgo: Elixir of Youth* (Capitola, CA: Botanica Press, 1991), p. 55.

12. P. L. Le Bars et al., A placebo-controlled, double-blind, randomized trial of an extract of Ginkgo biloba for dementia, *Journal of the American Medical Association*. 267, no. 16 (1997): 1327–32.

13. See note 1 above.

Chapter 10. The Side Effects—and How to Avoid Them

1. D. M. Warburton, Clinical psychopharmacology of Ginkgo biloba extract, in E. W. Funfgeld, ed., *Rokan— Ginkgo biloba* (New York: Springer-Verlag, 1988).

2. *Physicians' Desk Reference,* 51st ed. (New Jersey: Medical Economics Company, 1997), p. 2318.

3. E. Bruchert, S. E. Heinrich, and P. Ruf-Kohler, [Effects of LI 1370 on older patients with cerebral insufficiency. Multicenter double-blind study of German General Industrial Union], *Münchener Medizinische Wochenschrift* 133, Suppl. 1 (1991): S9–14.

4. S. M. Beckstrom-Sternberg and J. A. Duke, Chemicals and their biological activities in: Ginkgo biloba L. (Ginkoaceae), in *Phytochemeco Database* (U.S. Department of Agriculture, 1998).

5. L. E. Becker and G. B. Skipworth, Ginkgo-tree dermatitis, stomatitis, and proctitis, *Journal of the American Medical*

Association 231, no. 11 (1975): 1162–63; and R. R. Tomb, J. Foussereau, and Y. Sell, Mini-epidemic of contact dermatitis from ginkgo tree fruit (Ginkgo biloba L.), *Contact Dermatitis* 19, no. 4 (1988): 281–83.

6. American Botanical Council (trans.), *German Federal Commission E Monograph: Ginkgo* (1994), available online at www.herbalgram.org.

7. J. Rowin and S. L. Lewis, Spontaneous bilateral subdural hematomas associated with chronic Ginkgo biloba ingestion, *Neurology* 46, no. 6 (1996): 1775–76; and G. J. Gilbert, Ginkgo biloba [letter], *Neurology* 48, no. 4 (1997): 1137.

8. M. Rosenblatt and J. Mindel, Spontaneous hyphema associated with ingestion of Ginkgo biloba extract, *New England Journal of Medicine* 336, no. 15 (1997): 1108.

9. See J. Rowin and S. L. Lewis in note 7 above.

10. M. Odawara, A. Tamaoka, and K. Yamashita, Ginkgo biloba [letter], *Neurology* 48, no. 3 (1997): 789–90.

11. See G. J. Gilbert in note 7 above.

12. See note 8 above.

13. *Physicians' Desk Reference,* 51st ed. (New Jersey: Medical Economics Company, 1997), p. 2319.

14. See note 3 above.

Chapter 11. Growing and Harvesting Ginkgo

1. J. Blackadar, *The Ginkgo Page* (1998), online at: www.blackadar.com/ginkgo/

2. X. Y. Yu et al., Analysis of ginkgolide B from leaves of Ginkgo biloba L. by HPLC, *Chinese Journal of Pharmaceutical Analysis* 13, no. 3 (1993): 85–88.

3. D. Kustrak, Z. Males, and A. Sever, Pharmacobotanical investigation of Ginkgo biloba leaves, *Farmaceutski Glasnik* 51, no. 11 (1995): 291–302.

Appendix 1. Why This Book Is Cruelty-Free

1. American Anti-Vivisection Society, *AAVS Information: What Is Vivisection?* (1998), available online at www.aavs.org

2. W. Thacher, *Chimpanzees: Test Results That Don't Apply to Humans,* Physicians Committee for Responsible Medicine, informational pamphlet (1998); and W. Thacher, *Rats: Test Results That Don't Apply to Humans,* Physicians Committee for Responsible Medicine, informational pamphlet (1998). Both available online at www.pcrm.org

3. K. Sasaki et al., Bilobalide, a constituent of Ginkgo biloba L., potentiates drug-metabolizing enzyme activities in mice, *Research Communications in Molecular Pathology and Pharmacology* 96, no. 1 (1997): 45–56.

4. S. B. Hwang and M. H. Lam, Species difference in the specific receptors of platelet activating factor, *Biochemical Pharmacology* 35, no. 24 (1986): 4511–18.

5. Physicians Committee for Responsible Medicine, *Birth Defect Research: Why Animal Experiments Are Not the Answer,* PCRM informational pamphlet (1998), available online at www.pcrm.org

INDEX

About the Author

Jonathan Zuess, M.D., is a physician who has trained in both conventional and alternative medicine. His interest in natural medicine is a family tradition, stretching back many generations. After completing medical school, he did an internship in conventional medicine and a residency in psychiatry. He achieved one of the highest scores of all time on the United States Medical Licensing Exam and continued to score in the top one percent of residents in psychiatry and neurology in the United States and Canada. Aware of the limitations of conventional medicine, he went on to study a number of alternative therapies, including herbalism, nutrition, Asian medicine, and homeopathy. He is a member of the American Holistic Medical Association. He is the author of *The Natural Prozac Program: How to Use St. John's Wort, the Antidepressant Herb* (New York: Harmony Books, 1997), and *The Wisdom of Depression: A Guide to Understanding and Curing Depression Using Natural Medicine* (New York: Harmony Books, 1998). He is also an avid backpacker and has spent several months exploring remote wilderness areas in Australia. He practices medicine in Arizona.